DATE DUE

APR 1 8 1997	
OCT 2 2 1998	
SEP 27 1999	
2 9	
Van Island Reg due Jan 17/04	

BRODART   Cat. No. 23-221

Practising Nursing — Becoming Experienced

To my mother
Laura Margaret Smith Peach
whose own wisdom and valued experience
merits greater recognition

For Churchill Livingstone:

Editorial director: Mary Law
Project development editor: Dinah Thom
Copy editor: Anita Hible
Project manager: Valerie Burgess
Project controller: Pat Miller/Derek Robertson
Design direction: Judith Wright
Sales promotion executive: Hilary Brown

Practising Nursing – Becoming Experienced

Martha L. P. MacLeod RN BA MA PhD
Associate Professor, Nursing Programme
Faculty of Health and Human Sciences,
University of Northern British Columbia,
Prince George, B.C., Canada

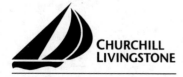
CHURCHILL
LIVINGSTONE

NEW YORK EDINBURGH LONDON MADRID MELBOURNE SAN FRANCISCO AND TOKYO 1996

CHURCHILL LIVINGSTONE
Medical Division of Pearson Professional Limited

Distributed in the United States of America by
Churchill Livingstone, 650 Avenue of the Americas, New
York, N.Y. 10011, and by associated companies, branches and
representatives throughout the world.

First published 1996

ISBN 0 443 05279 4

British Library Cataloguing in Publication Data
A catalogue record for this book is available from the British
Library.

Library of Congress Cataloging in Publication Data
A catalog record for this book is available from the Library of
Congress.

The
publisher's
policy is to use
**paper manufactured
from sustainable forests**

Produced by Longman Singapore Publishers (Pte) Ltd.
Printed in Singapore

Contents

Preface

When I first began this research, I intended to examine directly learning and experience in nursing. I knew from my background in adult education, that the conversation about learning is often eclipsed in our rush to talk about how we can facilitate learning through teaching. With few exceptions, our conversations about learning lack any mention of the integration of the bodily knowing that is basic to practising nursing well. Thus, in order to understand just how expertise develops it seemed important to take an indirect approach and to look at where experience and learning occur. Among nurses this is in the midst of nursing practice.

Patricia Benner pointed me in the direction of hermeneutic phenomenology — a research approach which probes in depth the lived experience of individuals, in this text the ward sisters' experience of nursing. This approach also enables background practices and meanings to come into view and readily allows insight into the bodily aspects of nurses' knowing and learning.

Hermeneutic phenomenology demands that the researcher takes an indirect approach to the study of a phenomenon. Interpretation is needed to unearth the phenomenon from the ground of experience. In my study, nursing practice readily came into view. I had to look much deeper, however, to see the character of learning and experience. My focus on the nature of everyday experience in nursing practice allowed me to move beyond a description of experience and practice to an ontological exploration of experiencing and practising nursing. Ontology is concerned with seeking an understanding of the nature and meaning of being itself. It is sometimes expressed through the question, 'What ways are there of "being in the world" '? It was through this ontological exploration that the nature of incidental or natural learning was revealed.

In the course of this research, and in the ensuing years, I have realized anew how important the context of our practices is in forming our understanding. This book is heavily influenced by several cultural contexts. The research builds on the work done by Patricia Benner in the United States. It was undertaken in Scotland by myself, a Canadian. I have had a unique opportunity to examine the language of nursing and to see how our practices, our language and our knowledge are formed within the contexts in which we work, study and learn. One of the challenges has been to translate nursing language, first so I could understand it, and second, so I could speak in a voice that bridged the cultures.

In this book, the excellent, experienced nurses whose practice was examined, are ward sisters. In the United Kingdom, many ward sisters are clinical experts despite mounting pressure for the role to become predominantly a managerial one. The excellent, experienced Ward Sisters in the study show clinical leadership that is integral to their managerial effectiveness. In the course of examining everyday practice, I have excavated some of the ground of clinical leadership.

I have referred to the study participants as Ward Sisters or 'the Sisters' throughout. Colleagues in

North America have sometimes found the term 'Sisters' to be disconcerting and have wondered if the nurses are also members of religious orders. They are not. I have not revised the term to 'charge nurses', 'nurse managers', or simply 'nurses' for several reasons. At the time of the study in the Scottish hospitals, the Ward Sisters were always referred to as 'Sister' by nurses, doctors, patients and other staff. The name 'Sister' carries with it a history of clinical leadership, knowledge and nursing authority. With the use of the word 'Sister' comes an inherent respect for the position that embraces the person. This authority and respect are enhanced when the person in the position is an excellent, experienced nurse.

The head nurses in my ongoing Canadian study are as experienced, excellent and respected as are the Scottish Sisters. It is notable, however, that the clinical and managerial authority of the Canadian head nurses is not as readily reflected in everyday language. For example, in Canadian hospitals doctors are referred to on the wards as 'Doctor', but the head nurses are referred to by their first names. Their authority and position are not automatically part of their naming. I have not yet explored the significance of this difference between the countries, but for me it points towards the importance of the names we use. As the Scottish nurses understood themselves and were understood by others to be ward sisters, it seems appropriate that I refer to them as the Sisters. I ask the forbearance of those readers for whom this term is not familiar.

As a nurse, a manager and an educator, I am aware that we often simplify practices and ideas in order that novices may learn them. In this book, the inherent complexity of nursing practice is revealed and new light is shed on understanding how people experience and learn. Experience and learning are shown to be complex and intertwined with the ongoing context in which they occur. Efforts to simplify the notions of experience and learning can too easily strip them of their context, and thus eliminate much of their meaning. In the rich descriptions of nursing practice, experience and learning, readers may find many points for fruitful discussion. I invite readers to enter into a dialogue with the nurses' experiences and my interpretations, and through that dialogue to find ways in which to bring their own learning and experience to light.

Northern British Columbia, 1996   M.L.P. MacL.

Acknowledgements

This book is based on my PhD thesis. The study was undertaken between 1986 and 1990 while I was on leave from the Nursing Division of St Boniface General Hospital, Winnipeg, Canada, and based at the Department of Nursing Studies at the University of Edinburgh. Sustained financial support from the St Boniface General Hospital Research Foundation and an Overseas Research Student Award from the Committee of Vice-Chancellors and Principals of the United Kingdom enabled me to delve more deeply into the meaning of experience, learning and expertise than might otherwise have been possible.

My supervisors, Kath Melia and Dai Hounsell, provided me with just the right measure of stimulation, challenge and support. From them, I have learned much about the value of clarity in thinking and in writing. Penny Prophit's encouragement in the early stages of this work was particularly appreciated. All three have helped me to learn many things that have wider application beyond the bounds of this project.

Colleagues have been tremendously supportive throughout the study and the development of this book. Steve Tilley's questions, careful reading and thoughtful challenges to my thinking have contributed immeasurably to the quality of this work. Philip Darbyshire's example, encouragement and gentle prodding have played a large role in my bringing the Sisters' voices to a wider audience. Even from a distance, both Steve and Philip continue to provide consistent moral support,

stimulating discussion and above all, laughter, when it is most needed. Nancy Diekelmann encouraged my scholarship throughout the study and continues to create a place to dwell and to expand my understanding of hermeneutics. I am indebted to Patricia Benner for her scholarship and encouragement. My colleagues at the University of Northern British Columbia have been most supportive and have taken on more themselves in order that I might finish the book. A sustaining force has been Jan Dick's enduring belief in the capacity of nurses to create a future for nursing that serves patients well.

From the outset, my husband, Tom, and children, Calum and Allie, have viewed this project as an adventure; they have done everything they could do to make it possible. To say that their support has been invaluable would be to trivialize the nature of their love and commitment. I indeed do know how lucky I am.

My greatest thanks go to the 10 Sisters in the study who shared themselves and their nursing practice with me most warmly and openly. I am privileged to have been able to work with them and to be able to tell about their practice and experience. Their interest and encouragement through the later phases of the research helped to sustain the momentum when it otherwise might have flagged. Their interest continues long-distance. I could not have hoped to have worked with a more professional, caring group of excellent practitioners.

Some of the material published in this book, particularly in Chapters 5 and 6, appeared in similar form as MacLeod M 1994 The everyday experience of nursing practice. In: Lathlean J, Vaughan B (eds) Unifying nursing practice and theory. Butterworth Heinemann, Oxford, pp 33–51. I am grateful to Butterworth Heinemann for their permission to use the material in this book.

Notations used in field notes and interview transcription

Field notes for each day were written onto the computer from notes taken hastily on the ward in a small notebook. For purposes of quotations in the text, I have made some minor stylistic changes:

- Where pertinent, the tense has been changed to the present tense.
- Sentence structure of some of my observations has been changed in a minor way; quotations taken at the time have not been altered.
- Minor changes which add explanation, such as a patient's name or diagnosis, or number of days postoperatively, have been made. They are enclosed by square brackets.

The interviews were transcribed verbatim, including all 'err's', 'um's' and facilitative sounds such as 'mm hmm', on the part of the interviewer. Where these sounds, repetitions and hesitations have not added to the meaning of the quotation, they have been omitted. Lengthy omissions are indicated by [...].

In the field notes and interview transcriptions, the following have been used:

1. :: :: Missed conversation in the field notes. The greater the number, the more of a gap. Each :: means a phrase or short sentence
2. [...] I have edited the field notes or interviews
3. ... Pause on the part of the speaker. The length of pause is indicated by the number of dots.
4. [words] Explanatory notes
5. (word) A response from other nurse present or the patient, e.g. (laughs)
6. italics My interpretative comments which were written at the time in the field notes
7. bold My emphasis
8. CAPS Speaker's emphasis

The references W4D2 etc. refer to the coding scheme for field notes and interviews, for example:

- W4D2–1.3 is Ward 4, Day 1 of the second visit, page 3 of the field notes.
- W4D2:3 is Ward 4, Day 2 of the first visit, page 3 of the field notes.
- Int. 7–2:3 is Interview 2 with Sister on Ward 7, page 3 of interview transcript.

1

Introduction

BACKGROUND TO THE STUDY

Over the last decade, we have become more aware that current ways of understanding learning only partially capture what happens in professionals' everyday practice. Excellent, experienced nurses talk about how they are learning all the time and readily acknowledge that their formal education marks only the beginning of learning their profession. They are not alone in their experience. Indeed, all of us, working day-by-day, experience a deepening of knowledge and an increase in our range of skills and abilities to manage an ever wider variety of situations. We all experience learning during our working day, even though we may not intend to learn. Often we do not attend directly to our learning. We take it for granted. This book is about this taken-for-granted, natural or incidental learning — learning in the midst of experience. The context is nursing.

Learning has long been studied within educational contexts, but learning that is independent of efforts to educate has received scant attention, even in the field of adult learning (Thomas 1986). Attempts to study informal and incidental learning in the workplace have focused directly on learning in the context of facilitating that learning, or improving worker and organizational productivity (Marsick & Watkins 1990, Senge 1990). This book will show that in order to gain an in-depth understanding of incidental learning, the practice and experience within which learning occurs must receive direct attention. Throughout the book it becomes apparent that what we take for granted comes to light only when experience itself is excavated. Thus, the book takes as its starting point and focus, the everyday experience of 'excellent, experienced' nurses.

In looking at experience, the book operates on two levels. At first glance, the depiction of nurses' everyday experience and the context of that experience, nursing practice, would be of interest only to nurses. The discussion however, does not just remain with an ontic depiction of nursing experience and practice. It goes further, showing how nurses engage in practising nursing and experiencing their practice. It is at this level, where I directly address questions of experience, learning and the development of expertise among professionals, that this exploration of nurses' everyday experience can be considered as a paradigm case in the study of organizations and of workplace learning.

Nurses are not alone in their experience of organizational and system changes that are creating new demands to extend and deepen their knowledge and skills. The changes in the skills structure within Western societies are reflected in private and public sector organizations alike. In acute care hospitals, it could be said that the need for nursing expertise has never been greater. The 'inexorable continuation of the trend towards shorter hospital stays' (Moores 1989), together with an ageing population, changes in patterns of illness, rapid advances in technology and the accompanying changes in medical practice, have meant that patients in hospitals have increasingly complex care requirements. These complex care requirements are to be met within a health care system that is undergoing considerable structural and organizational change. To respond to such demands with 'ingenuity and the development of innovative practices' (Auld 1988 p 85), the development, support and retention of experienced nurses with clinical expertise is critical. This is perhaps more easily said than done, particularly when we understand so little about the nature of experience and the development of expertise in nursing practice. It is complicated by the fact that so little is known about the learning that occurs in the midst of ongoing, everyday activities.

This book is based on my doctoral research study in which I explore the nature of everyday experience in nursing practice with a view to gaining an understanding of how that everyday experience contributes to the development of nursing expertise. The participants in this interpretative study were 10 surgical ward sisters in two Scottish teaching hospitals who were considered by their nursing managers to be 'excellent, experienced' surgical nurses.

This study stemmed from a personal interest as well as a professional need. As head of a school of continuing education in a large Canadian teaching hospital I was involved in the development of educational programmes to meet the need for nurses trained for advanced clinical practice in specialty areas. In the course of planning for curriculum and organizational changes, I was intrigued by the commonsense knowledge of the teachers and head nurses (ward sisters) concerning the level of experience required by nurses to manage certain patient care situations. Some curriculum and organizational decisions were based on this commonsense knowledge. I began to realize how little understanding we have of the nature of everyday experience. Compared to experience which is a part of formal educational endeavours, everyday experience in the course of working as a nurse has been little valued. It also has received scant attention in the research literature.

Everyday experience merits in-depth examination for several reasons. First, there is a dearth of formal knowledge about the substance of nursing practice, what Meleis (1987) calls 'the business of nursing'. The substance of nursing lies in those caring practices which help people '... in the performance of those activities contributing to health, or its recovery (or to a peaceful death) that they would perform unaided if they had the necessary strength, will, or knowledge' (Henderson 1966). Such caring practices are often difficult to articulate because of their complexity and their reliance upon the context for meaning. An exploration of the knowledge and skills of experienced practitioners allows the practices to be revealed (McFarlane 1977, Benner 1984). As I will argue later, most studies focus on particular aspects of nursing practice; the full complexity of practice only comes to light in the ongoing context of everyday experience.

The second reason for an in-depth consideration of everyday experience is its relationship to the development of clinical competence. Everyday experience in clinical nursing practice is considered essential to the development of knowledge and skills because of the practice-based nature of the nursing profession. Experience in practice is necessary for learning, not only for students, but also for the ongoing development of expertise. A certain level of experience in a clinical area is often a prerequisite for entry into a post-basic course or for consideration for a more senior nursing position. However, despite the commonsense knowledge that experience accompanies learning and the development of expertise in a field, the link between them is relatively unexplored.

Several studies have examined the learning which occurs through experience in clinical practice. Lathlean et al's (1986) evaluation of a programme for newly registered nurses is not untypical. They delineated two different kinds of experience in clinical practice: *experience per se* (i.e. that which happened merely as a result of working as a registered nurse regardless of the particular environment) and *experience with specific conditions* or features which facilitated the learning, some of which existed by design (e.g. working alongside a highly skilled ward sister on a number of pre-arranged shifts) and some by accident (e.g. caring for someone with a rare disease who happened to be admitted to the ward) (p 59).

This distinction between 'experience per se' and 'experience with specific conditions' is an interesting one. The authors suggest that newly registered nurses learn more productively through specific kinds of experience. Indeed, educational structures and programmes are designed to give nurses specific, and often guided, clinical experience. In agreement with Lathlean et al (1986), Robinson & Elkan (1989) suggest that the two traditional methods through which learning takes place, 'experience' and 'role modelling', have their limitations: they are likely to reinforce the status quo, irrespective of the quality of the care provided; they are restricted in their applicability to the present role; and they rely upon qualities in newly registered nurses which not all newly registered nurses have, such as an ability to identify when they need help. While this argument is well taken, it embodies a certain

contradiction when extended, as it often is, to the education of experienced practitioners (cf. Working Party on Continuing Education 1981).

The contradiction centres on the fact that practitioners extend and deepen their skills and knowledge without educational interventions. It is acknowledged that staff nurses and ward sisters gain their knowledge and skills largely through everyday practice: 'They learn mainly from personal experience and from observation...' (Working Party on Continuing Education 1981). While it is properly argued that educational programmes, particularly patient-centred ones, are critical to the development of sufficient numbers of nursing practitioners with the advanced levels of skills necessary to provide the required level of care (Henderson 1980, Dick 1983, Pembrey 1989), it cannot be denied that some nurses develop expertise in their day-to-day practice, sometimes without the benefit of such formal education programmes. At the same time, it is recognized that some staff nurses and ward sisters advance the development of nursing knowledge through their ongoing practice. As Dick (1983) says about the excellent practising nurse: 'She is scholarly in the sense that she knows what questions to ask to resolve problems in nursing care and to advance nursing practice'. McFarlane (1977) reminds us of our impressions of the wisdom of experienced ward sisters, 'If we could only catch their wisdom and write it down we would have a rich feast of concepts of nursing practice'. I will be arguing in the following chapters that we should not discount ongoing, moment-by-moment experience because of its importance in the development of expertise.

Before moving on to an overview of the chapters, it may be useful to explain how I came to study 'excellent, experienced' ward sisters. When I first came to Scotland, I sought to study 'expert' nurses, as Benner (1984) had done. Early discussions at the University and with nurses in clinical practice indicated to me that the word 'expert' was an unfamiliar one, particularly in the context of a bedside nurse. I was questioned countless times about why I wished to do the research in Scotland. Typical comments were: 'The funding is so bad, all nurses can do is physical task care', 'Where will you find experts?

The good ones don't stay in nursing for long', 'But American nursing is 10 years ahead of us!' These comments intrigued me, as nurses from the UK generally have a reputation in Canadian hospitals for being good, thoughtful, patient-centred bedside nurses. When I met with the Directors of Nursing Services in the two hospitals in which I conducted my study, they agreed that the word 'expert' was ambiguous, but they readily identified 10 'excellent, experienced' surgical nurses, eight of whom were ward sisters and two of whom undertook ward sister duties. Appendix 1 details the research approach, methods and the selection process for the Sisters.

Language differences are an inescapable part of this study. One of the complicating factors in any discussion of nursing practice and experience in the UK by a Canadian is the way in which the English language is used. The weather provides a fine example of this. In Edinburgh, a day in which the temperature reached 23° Celsius was described on the radio as a 'scorcher', whereas in Winnipeg it would need to be well over 30° Celsius before 'scorcher' would be used. Although many countries share nursing terms and notions, these terms have different meanings or nuances of meanings within each country. The words are the same and we therefore often assume that the meanings are the same when they are not. I hope that in this study I have adequately captured the meanings in the Sisters' practices and experiences, and that the differences in culture and language have uncovered as much as they have hidden in this exploration of everyday experience.

CHAPTER PREVIEW

The structure of the book is as follows. Chapter 2 begins with an exploration of how experience has been depicted in the learning and experience literature. This literature, drawn upon extensively in nursing education, proposes a number of ways in which to understand experience and the learning which accompanies it. I suggest that much of the literature treats experience as if it were non-problematic. The focus remains on learning and its facilitation. I argue that such a focus is inadequate and in order to understand experience in its complexity, it must be examined directly. The development of expertise forms the second part of the chapter. I suggest that the Dreyfus Model of Skill Acquisition (Dreyfus & Dreyfus 1986) provides a useful perspective on expertise because of its attention to the contextual nature of knowledge and the connection between experience and the development of expertise.

Chapter 3 details the various approaches which have been applied to the study of nursing practice. As the participants in the study are ward sisters, I pay particular attention to studies of the ward sister. I argue here that the approach used by Benner (1984, 1985, 1994) captures the complexity of nursing practice missing from other studies and discuss the merits of adopting a similar approach.

In Chapters 4, 5, 6, and 7, themes which emerged from the analysis of the Sisters' accounts and my observations of their practice are discussed. In Chapter 4, the problematic nature of experience is addressed. Rather than being static and spatial, everyday experience was found to be elusive, complex and continually changing. Experience is not something discrete, separate and private: it is in continuous interplay with the Sisters' ongoing practices.

Chapter 5 describes what I understand the Sisters to be doing as they practice. I suggest that they help individual patients towards recovery, and in order to do this, they make the ward work. Their practice is seen to be patient-centred, complex, goal-directed and multifaceted.

In Chapter 6, the inextricably intertwined process through which the Sisters practise nursing — noticing, understanding and acting — is described. I suggest in this chapter that the quality of this process contributes to their expertise in nursing. In Chapter 7, I argue that this process of practising is also the process of developing expertise. The various ways in which the Sisters learn in everyday practice are explored.

In the final chapter, the themes are extended to a discussion of 'being attuned to experience'. I argue that it is through this process that the Sisters, these 'excellent experienced' nurses, practise and develop expertise. I suggest that the 'knowing' which develops through being attuned to experience is more complex than is conventionally depicted in the theory/practice discussions in nursing. Likewise it is argued that the customary separations of action/reflection and learning/experience are less useful for understanding the development of expertise in everyday experience than is the more subtle process of 'being attuned to experience'. I suggest that by looking anew at everyday experience in nursing practice, the value of that experience and practice, and their contribution to the development of expertise, will be revealed.

The chapter concludes with a discussion of the implications of rethinking our current views of learning and experience for nursing practice, for the education of nurses, and for nursing's professional aspirations. While the findings of the study cannot be directly extrapolated to learners in undergraduate or post-graduate programmes, the discussion explores ways in which new understandings of learning and experience can influence nursing education and professional development programmes as well as nursing organizations and worklife.

RESEARCH APPROACH AND METHOD

Before proceeding, it is necessary to give the reader some idea of how the research was undertaken. The quality of interpretative phenomenological research can be assessed in part, by considering its coherence and depth. Appendix 1 details both the research approach and method. For those who may wish to judge the study by seeing how the interpretations were reached, and for those who may wish to conduct a similar study, the Appendix provides in-depth discussion of the decisions I made and the actions I took. For those who do not find such discussions particularly interesting or pertinent, the following will provide sufficient working knowledge of the study to place the ensuing discussion in context.

I approached the study from a stance of interpretative or hermeneutic phenomenology (Heidegger 1962, Gadamer 1975, Ricoeur 1978, Benner 1994), with a goal of understanding the everyday experience of being a nurse. Phenomenology is concerned with the meaning of experience; hermeneutics is an 'attempt to make clear, to make sense of an object of study' (Taylor 1971). Using hermeneutic phenomenology, new light can be shed on our taken-for-granted, background practices. This philosophical approach helped me to attend explicitly to the complexities of experience and learning in the midst of ongoing work situations.

The Ward Sisters worked on a variety of surgical wards in the two teaching hospitals, including general surgery, ENT, gynaecology, thoracic surgery, and urology. During 11 months of field work I 'shadowed' the Ward Sisters and interviewed them three times each, and once as a group. In the interviews, I asked the nurses to describe experiences in their practice and to make links between past and current experiences. The field notes arising from the participant observation and interview transcripts provided the text for a hermeneutic interpretation.

Two principles were touchstones throughout the research. First, my attention was focused on the nurse-in-practice, not on the nurse removed from a context, nor on the context without the nurse. Second, I tried to keep close to experience, to continually ask while in the field and during interpretation, 'What does this mean about experience?'. During the interpretation process, I sought to bring to light the meanings and relational qualities of everyday, taken-for-granted practices. An understanding of nursing practice, experience and learning emerged and I have endeavoured to create a credible, robust interpretation. In keeping with the tenets of hermeneutic interpretation, the reader participates in determining the quality of the research and the interpretation. Moving between excerpts of data and discussion, the reader enters into the hermeneutic circle of understanding and interpretation, and judges whether the report is indeed 'a plausible story' (Strong 1979 p 250), and 'one that makes theoretical sense' (Silverman 1989).

2

Experience and the development of expertise

INTRODUCTION

Experience, as a word and a phenomenon, is notoriously slippery. Although it is commonly understood and taken-for-granted in everyday conversation, it becomes elusive when it is directly examined. The various shades of meaning of the word *experience* give a hint of its complexity. The Shorter Oxford Dictionary describes experience variously as: being consciously the subject of a state or condition; the observation of facts or events; the state of having been in everyday life and, in addition, the effects of having been so engaged. To further complicate matters, to experience is to have experience. Generally speaking, experience refers to something which has gone before as well as to action ongoing in the present.

In scientific and philosophical writing, the debate about experience has been substantial and wide-ranging. Experience has been depicted as an objective phenomenon, a subjective phenomenon and a phenomenon concerned with being-in-the-world. The nature of experience is closely tied to what it means to be a person, living and being in the world, and because of this it may not be possible to obtain either a clear or unitary picture of experience.

Before we begin to address the question of the nature of everyday experience for experienced nurses, it may be helpful to look at how experience is depicted within two different but related areas of knowledge which are extensively drawn upon by nurses. The first area concerns learning from experience — what is often called experiential learning. The second concerns knowledge and its relationship to the development of expertise in nursing. By examining these perspectives, we will see how current ways of understanding experience and learning fail to adequately account for how nurses experience their ongoing, everyday practice and how they develop expertise.

EXPERIENCE AND LEARNING

Over the past few decades, there has been a plethora of research on experiential learning. Most of the research has been about 'deliberate' learning experiences (Tough 1979). Incidental or natural learning, learning which happens incidentally in the midst of other activities, has received lesser attention.

A number of experiential learning models have arisen from studies of deliberate learning. They are important to consider because they have gained prominence in educational and workplace movements, for example, 'the learning organization' and 'reflective practice'. With few exceptions, the models' conceptions of experience, learning and reflection have been treated non-problematically. As we will see in subsequent chapters, particularly Chapters 4 and 6, experience and the process of experiencing are more problematic and complex than the models portray. Before turning to deliberate learning and to research that explores natural or incidental learning, it may be useful to briefly consider how experience is viewed in definitions of experiential learning.

Experiential learning is a term that is variously used to depict ways in which learning and experience are linked. Sometimes it is used to describe the form of education as well as the learning which occurs (McGill & Weil 1990). In a survey of educators involved in experiential learning (Henry 1989), the minority view was that all learning was experiential. More frequently, experiential learning was considered to be a sequence of stages of which experience was but one. The educators taking this view believed that, '. . . experience alone [is] not enough, to count as experiential learning: the 'experiencer' has to consciously realize the *value*

of that experience' (p 28). This view, of the need to bring experience to conscious awareness in order for learning to occur, is a recurring one. It is based on an underlying assumption that experience and learning are separate entities. This position, I will argue, reflects a particular, but predominant view of experience which merits re-examination.

Deliberate learning experiences

'Deliberate learning' experiences are experiences planned with learning in mind. They are usually part of educational programmes, either inside the classroom or in the workplace, but also may be part of self-directed learning projects which can occur in any part of a person's life (Tough 1979). In any case, the goal of the situation is learning and 'learners' are aware that they are learning. Models and theories of experiential learning have been developed from deliberate learning situations, particularly those in which the goal of learning is more than merely the acquisition of information. The view of learning and experience expressed in these models and theories permeates the nursing literature, particularly the literature on learning or developing expertise.

Experiential learning models

There are eight key models or theories in the field of experiential learning: those of Lewin (1952), Revans (1980), Kolb (1984), Jarvis (1987a, 1987b), Argyris & Schön (1974), Boud et al (1985), Mezirow (1981, 1990, 1994) and Freire (1970). Common to all is the centrality of concrete experience as the source and testing ground for learning. With the exception of Mezirow (1994) and Freire (1970), all are cyclical in nature, with some form of feedback loop in which learning from one experience influences the next. Although the models are grounded in experience, the theorists do not excavate that ground. The focus of the models is on learning, particularly learning which restructures perceptions of situations and oneself (Boydell 1976). Experience is viewed, for the most part, as an entity to be used or developed. The models or theories generally can be categorized as action learning models (Lewin, Revans, Kolb, Jarvis) or as models of reflection (Argyris & Schön, Boud et al, Mezirow, Freire).

Action learning models: The action learning models are characterized by several-stage, systematic and rational processes. Concrete experience is the ground for learning and is usually identified as one of the stages in the model.

Lewin's model of action research: One of the first experiential learning models, Lewin's (1952) model of action research and laboratory training, is described as a social learning and problem-solving process. The model, developed from work with groups, emphasizes the importance of concrete experience to validate and test abstract concepts. Experience is considered to provide a robust source for concepts and a context for testing them, but it is not explored in any detail. Lewin's focus is on the social field and on the interplay between the subjective (perception) and the objective (action). Lewin identified four stages of learning: concrete experience, observations and reflections, the formation of abstract concepts and generalizations, and the testing of the implications of concepts in new situations (see Figure 2.1). These have continued to be the major stages of experiential learning models.

Revans' theory of action learning: Revans' theory of 'action learning' (1980) was developed in the context of management education programmes where managers (learners) learn to solve problems in real-life situations. Like Lewin, Revans suggests

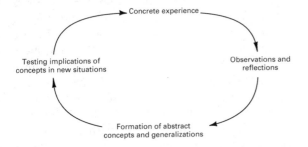

Figure 2.1 Lewinian experiential learning model. Reproduced from Kolb D 1984 Experiential learning: experience as the source of learning and development Reprinted by permission of Prentice-Hall Inc., Englewood Cliffs, NJ.

that learning is an adaptive process of behavioural change involving a circular learning process. He links action learning to the scientific method.

Kolb's experiential learning model: Kolb's (1984) experiential learning model remains the most widely-used experiential learning model in nursing. As it is so influential, it is explored in some detail here. This model was developed from Kolb's work in management development programmes and stems from the traditions of Dewey, Piaget and Lewin in cognitive and social psychology. Learning is viewed as a process of human development, 'the process whereby knowledge is created through the transformation of experience' (p 38). The model centres on the interconnection of knowledge and learning. Knowledge is not considered to be an independent entity to be acquired or transmitted: it is 'a transformation process being continuously created and re-created' (p 38). The transformation process occurs in the interplay between expectation and experience.

In Kolb's view, experience is where learning begins and ends. Experience is concrete: something that happens to a person and in which a person is involved. Citing Dewey (1938), Kolb considers experience to be a transactional relationship between the person and the environment, between the internal or subjective and the external or objective. According to Kolb, however, experience in itself is not enough. It must be both grasped and transformed, a process which is most frequently depicted by a four-stage cycle (Kolb 1984, Kolb & Lewis 1986).

In the cycle, which is much like the Lewinian cycle in Figure 2.1, immediate, concrete experience is the basis for observation and reflection (the grasping of experience through apprehension and comprehension). In turn, these observations are 'assimilated into an idea or theory from which new implications for action can be deduced' (Kolb & Lewis 1986). This is intention, the creation of concepts which integrate the observations into logically sound theories. Next, these theories are used to make decisions and to solve problems: through extension new experiences are created. Thus, not only are learning and experience separate and then integrated, but also action and reflection are considered to be disparate entities.

While Kolb emphasizes the importance of experience, he spends very little time examining what he means by it. The depiction of experience as a series of discrete entities, happening in real life, is consistent with both the conceptual roots and source of the model, i.e. meaningful experiences discussed in management classes. This very specific conception of experience is often overlooked when the model is extrapolated to other situations.

In Kolb's discussion of facilitating experiential learning, the separation of learning and experience extends to the place where each may occur. 'Immediate, concrete experiences that occur outside the classroom serve to arouse observation, prompt reflection and spur action' (Kolb & Lewis 1986). Even though Kolb describes learning as an adaptive process in which individuals adapt to their social and physical environments, he does not develop the link with everyday, ongoing experience to any great extent. His description of the experiential learning process remains somewhat removed from the everyday, moment-by-moment flow of living.

Jarvis: learning in the social context: Citing the confines on Kolb's model created by the narrow source of experiences, Jarvis (1987a) criticizes the model for its limited recognition of the social realm, for its simplicity, particularly in light of the complexity of experience and learning in natural situations, and for the fact that it overlooks the issue of meaning in learning. Jarvis goes on to create a new, complex model from data on 'learning experiences' provided by educators in workshops on adult learning and teaching.

Perhaps because of the source of these data, Jarvis explores experience to a greater extent than do other action learning theorists. Although Jarvis (1987a) recognizes that 'experience in the real world is a very complex phenomenon' (p 26), and identifies 16 different kinds of experience, the complexity is not evident in his descriptions. He consistently describes experience as an entity 'which is itself socially constructed and received through a variety of senses' (p 84). As an entity, experience contains sense data which can be used in learning (p 149). Separated from experience is reflection, which occurs retrospectively upon experience.

Jarvis' separation of experience and reflection is consistent with his distinction between an experience and a learning experience. He follows on from Berger & Luckmann (1967) in distinguishing between a situation and experience. He holds that '...it is the subjective definition of the situation which creates the experience and potentially leads to learning' (Jarvis 1987a p 70). Jarvis describes the connection between the individual and his/her situation as an interplay between the subjective and objective, where the individual imposes subjective, socially constructed meanings upon objective, socially defined situations.

This separation of subject and object is carried further. Jarvis holds that learning results from a disjunction between the individual's biography 'and the socio-cultural milieu in which the experience occurs' (p 79). Jarvis contends that learning occurs when the individual confers meaning upon situations. As some experiences may be meaningless to the individual, learning can be prevented. While Jarvis extends Kolb's work to include a broader range of situations, and delineates a variety of ways in which learning can emerge from experience, he, like Kolb, treats experience as a non-problematic, static entity.

Models of reflection: Reflection is at the centre of four other prominent theories of experiential learning: Boud et al (1985), Argyris & Schön (1974), Mezirow (1981, 1990, 1994) and Freire (1970). For Boud et al, experience is the starting point and the object of reflection; for Argyris & Schön, experience is the source and testing ground of theories of action which are formulated during periods of reflection; Mezirow considers experience to be the ground for transformative learning; Freire describes experience as the context for educational *praxis*.

Boud's model of reflection: Boud et al (1985) define experience as a static, though perhaps complex, entity. Even though an initial experience may be 'quite complex and is constituted of a number of particular experiences within it' (p 19), it is essentially a source of data. The data come from the experience: 'the total response of a person to a situation or event: what he or she thinks, feels, does and concludes at the time and immediately thereafter' (p 18). Unlike Jarvis, Boud et al do not discern between learning experiences and non-learning experiences. However, they focus on learning experiences in deliberate learning endeavours which can be described and recalled by the participants as discrete entities.

In a later article, Boud & Walker (1990) focus more directly on experience itself and depict experience in somewhat less static terms. They describe experience as 'the situation as it is known and lived by the learner' (p 62) and on-going experience as 'a continuing, complex series of interactions between the learner and the learning milieu, unified by reflective processes...' (p 66). The learning milieu is considered to be a social, psychological and material environment. Two aspects of the interactions are described as noticing and intervening. Reflection, a normal ongoing process, allows the learner to process what is perceived in a situation and becomes the basis of new knowledge and further action. Boud & Walker (1990) conclude that 'it is the learner's involvement with the event that constitutes the learning experience' (p 78). It is notable that even in an on-going experience, at the moment of reflection, the learner is, by definition, detached from the experience. Thus, even in Boud et al's refined model, the dichotomy between experience and reflection serves to emphasize reflection because the processing of experience is considered to be the key to learning.

Mezirow's theory of transformative learning: Mezirow (1981, 1990, 1994) situates his theory of transformative learning in the broader context of Habermas' (1984) theory of communicative action. He suggests that there are two learning domains (instrumental and communicative), and an emancipatory learning process in which critical reflection plays an important part. Individuals, groups and collectives can engage in a process of transformation by critically reflecting upon the presuppositions of uncritically assimilated meaning schemes and perspectives that come from experience. 'Learning is defined as the social process of construing and appro-

priating a new or revised interpretation of the meaning of one's experience as a guide to action' (Mezirow 1994 pp 222–223). Again, experience is relatively unexamined in Mezirow's formulation: he concentrates on the meaning structures and on processes and phases of reflection which enable what he calls, 'perspective transformation'.

Freire's process of conscientization: An approach which is increasingly being mentioned in discussions on reflection, learning and experience is that of Paulo Freire (1970). Freire describes a process of *conscientization*, a praxis — a fusing of action and reflection. Experience, in Freirean discourse, is linked to societal experience and serves as the basis for educational praxis. Reflection is contextualized in experience. Freire does not dwell on learning itself, but rather focuses on the educative and transformative nature of conscientization. Freire acknowledges the complexity of experience but does not concentrate on the nature of experience itself.

Argyris & Schön: theory of action perspective: Unlike the other experiential learning models, Argyris & Schön's (1974) 'theory of action perspective' does not address experience directly. Instead Argyris & Schön describe a fairly mechanistic, behavioural world in which actors design their behaviour for interpersonal action and hold theories for so doing. They suggest that theories operate at two levels: espoused theories which people use to explain or justify behaviour, and theories-in-use which are implicit in people's patterns of spontaneous behaviour with others. Argyris & Schön describe two models of theories-in-use:

1. Model I, in which existing patterns are maintained.
2. Model II, in which the values and assumptions underlying existing patterns are explored and changed towards a more open, effective behavioural world.

They contend that most people's theories-in-use are of the Model I variety although their espoused theories may differ.

According to Argyris & Schön, learning occurs in a single-loop or double-loop pattern. Single-loop learning retains the status quo; the more reflective double-loop learning involves questioning underlying assumptions and values. Not surprisingly, Argyris & Schön argue for an increase of Model II action and double-loop learning. In this theory, there is separation of the person (actor) and the (behavioural) world. Experience, when it is touched on, is described in terms of a subjective phenomenon. This depiction of experience is maintained in the authors' later works (Schön 1987, Argyris 1993).

Experiential learning models: a summary: Overall, the picture of experience and learning painted by the experiential learning models is somewhat stark and compartmentalized. Experience, learning, reflection and action are described as being distinct and are connected in specific, sequential and circular ways. Although experience forms the ground for each of the models, with the exception of Jarvis' model and Boud & Walker's later work, it remains unexamined. Notable in most of the models is the independence of the individual actor and the distinction of experience as a purely subjective or purely objective phenomenon. Mezirow and Freire are somewhat more successful in acknowledging the complex and situated nature of experience, but they, too, leave experience for others to examine in depth.

The experience of learners in the classroom

Classroom experience and learning in higher education have a long history of research attention. Much of the research is of marginal interest here because it deals with intellectual development such as reading, writing and learning from lectures (e.g. Marton et al 1984). There are, however, insights afforded to the question of the nature of experience by a few phenomenological studies that attend to learners' experiences in university level courses.

Taylor (1986, 1987), Griffin (1987) and Chené (1985), in their studies of students in adult learning programmes, illustrated that when people considered their learning, they intermixed their experiences within and outwith the programmes. Additionally, Taylor's (1987) study revealed some of the overlooked

dimensions of learning experiences: the emotional nature of learning, the role of intuition, the relational quality of learning and the political dimension of learning. Denis & Richter (1987) have included intuitive learning in their understanding of experiential learning, as has Griffin (1987).

Griffin's (1987) notion of basic learning processes, 'inner happenings or experiences the learner has when engaged in learning' (p 210), is an important one. The characteristics of learning processes reveal something of Griffin's view of the active and changing nature of learning experiences: they are denoted by verbs; the action is within the learner; the process happens over time; only the learner knows what he or she is experiencing. A strength of Griffin's approach is her focus on the range of experience related to learning. A drawback is that she maintains the view of the subjective person within an objective world because she considers experience to be wholly within the learner.

Diekelmann (1989, 1992, 1993), Rather (1992) and MacLeod (1995) present a relational view of experience in their interpretative phenomenological studies of nursing students' experience. Themes such as 'learning as evaluation' (Diekelmann 1989), 'being well taught as experiencing structure' (MacLeod 1995) and 'nursing as a way of thinking' (Rather 1992) illustrate the intersubjective and contextual nature of the students' experience. Experience in these studies does not reside solely in the learner, nor is the world presented solely as an objective reality. The view of experience which emerges is relational, the experience of students in the context of educational programmes.

These few studies paint a more complex picture of experience than do the experiential learning models; the boundaries between experience and learning are much less clear-cut. However, with the exception of the studies of Diekelmann, MacLeod and Rather, learning continues to be the primary focus of the research, whilst experience remains in the background as a source and a backdrop. This is understandable given that the research subjects are intentional learners in educational programmes.

Workplace learning experience

A very different picture of learning and experience is painted by the various studies of educational experience in workplace settings. Studies such as those by Atkinson (1981), Moore (1986), Melia (1987) and those compiled by Geer (1972), illuminate the organizational and social processes which influence the experiences of learners such as medical students, nursing students and barbers. Clearly illuminated are the activities and constraints of the work milieu as well as the situational learning which is required of the learners. Although the starting point in these studies is the experience of the learners, the analysis quickly moves away into the underlying social processes and dimensions of the learning situations. The experiencing person and the nature of experience move into the background to allow the social environment to come firmly into view.

Organizational learning is receiving increasing attention in sociology, management and adult education literature. Indeed, the learning organization has been described as the successful organization of the future (Senge 1990, Watkins & Marsick 1993). Many of the studies of organizational learning have provided insights into individual and group learning in organizations by building on the work of the experiential learning theorists (Argyris & Schön 1974, Revans 1980, Kolb 1984). In the same way that these theorists have overlooked experience in their focus on learning, so has the research on organizational learning concentrated almost exclusively on learning and its facilitation. Organizational issues, problems and actions serve as the context and impetus for learning. Experience itself has received scant attention.

Incidental learning experience

Incidental or natural learning, learning which occurs in the midst of other, ongoing activities, has had a relatively short history of direct research attention. With notable exceptions (Marsick & Watkins 1990, Watkins & Marsick 1992), studies of incidental learning focus more directly on the nature of experience, and characteristically, they present a complex and dynamic view of experience.

Learning in the midst of managerial work

Burgoyne & Stuart (1976), Burgoyne & Hodgson (1983) and Davies & Easterby-Smith (1984) were among the first to show how managers in the United Kingdom learn in the midst of their everyday work. Their findings are echoed in the seminal studies of US managers by McCall, Lombardo & Morrison (1988) and by Van Velsor & Hughes (1990). Just as nursing students said they learned most in clinical practice (Melia 1987), the managers in these studies asserted that they learned most managerial skills from 'natural' experiential sources. The managers distinguished between learning and development. Learning concerned short-term gains and was picked up gradually over time, whereas development meant acquiring greater competence over a longer period of time and was linked to promotion.

Concentrating on what the manager picks up in moment-by-moment work, Burgoyne & Hodgson (1983) identified three stages of learning. Notable amongst the five processes identified in the second stage was the gradual and tacit change in orientation or attitude which occurred on the basis of cumulative experience. It is on this point — the gradual and cumulative nature of experience and the resultant change in outlook — that the results of Burgoyne & Hodgson's study diverge most from Kolb's (1984) and Argyris & Schön's (1974) experiential learning models. Although Burgoyne & Hodgson do not themselves make this connection, this divergence could be related to the static notion of experience conceptualized in the experiential learning models as compared to the moment-by-moment experience of a normal workflow.

Davies & Easterby-Smith (1984) found that development primarily came from being in new situations, for which the managers had responsibility and had thus to take action. Success led to increased confidence and the willingness to develop further. This study highlights the influence of the organization on the individual's experience.

Lessons learned by managers in the course of their experience were identified by McCall et al (1988) and Van Velsor & Hughes (1990) in their respective studies of men and women managers. McCall et al (1988) noted that the lessons 'must be dug out of complex, confusing, ambiguous situations . . . . The lessons are associated with particular experiences, and draw their meaning from that context' (p 9). A study of veteran managers in a variety of fields (Akin 1991a) reveals the powerful transformative nature of learning experiences. The studies clearly show that engagement in the learning experience is sparked by the need to know and a sense of role.

As McCall et al, Van Velsor & Hughes and Akin show, when the complexity of experience and the interconnection of learning and experience is the focus of study, a different language and set of actions for learning emerge. Akin (1991b) notes that the examination of learning experiences points out how our current language is ill-suited for talking about learning in experience. New metaphors that capture the context of the organizational experiences are needed.

Time and the situation in incidental learning

The influences of time and the situation in incidental learning were important findings in Rossing & Russell's (1987) and Rossing's (1991) studies of informal incidental learning among community volunteers. Forty individuals involved in community problem-solving groups were asked to recall experiences which may have contributed to their existing beliefs about effective functioning of community groups. Interestingly, the individuals had difficulty recalling specific events and making discrete connections between events and the learning derived from them. Situational factors were an important part of the learning instances: most happened in a person's early experiences with the group and few were recent or current. Like Burgoyne & Hodgson (1983), McCall et al (1988) and Van Velsor & Hughes (1990), many beliefs were traced to a gradual accumulation of experiences rather than to specific events. Rossing (1991) contends that the reflective

observation and experiential action stages of Kolb's (1984) model were rarely described by the participants. He suggests that these stages do not seem to be necessary for learning to occur.

The interplay of past and present

Quite a different perspective on experience and learning from experience is afforded by two studies (Gray-Snelgrove 1982, Hasselkus & Ray 1988) which consider both the past and ongoing experience of caregivers. Hasselkus & Ray studied caregivers of the frail elderly in the community whilst Gray-Snelgrove studied adult children caring for parents dying of cancer. The view of experience emerging from both studies is one of a complex phenomenon which is tied up with the meaning of ongoing activities. Although both studies reveal learning to be embedded in the ongoing situation and to be happening continuously, they diverge sharply in their descriptions of learning.

From their ethnographic interviews of family caregivers, Hasselkus & Ray identify six patterns of informal learning. They contend that these patterns of learning correspond to Schön's (1983) description of professional knowing, 'reflection-in-action'. Thus they suggest that the caregivers learned informally as they cared for their family members and that they carried out 'a reflective conversation with the situation as they named the things they would attend to and framed the context in which they would attend to them' (p 37).

Addressing the issue of time in experience and building herself into the research process, Gray-Snelgrove (1982) takes a unique approach to the issues of experience and learning. To study ongoing 'experiencing' as well as the meaning in past experience, she engaged in a joint exploration with individuals who were caring for a dying parent, and shared her own experiences in the course of the interviews. A hermeneutic analysis revealed the structure and dynamics of the meanings of caregiving and sharing experiences, seen in the context of time. Of particular interest are Gray-Snelgrove's conclusions about the ways in which talking helps people to grasp their pre-reflective knowing. Experience in this study is shown to be an interplay between past and present, and to be ever changing in the present. Rather than a subjective phenomenon, experience is shown to be intersubjective, and linked to meanings arising between people in specific situations.

Summary

Even in a field devoted to the consideration of experience and the learning which accompanies it, the nature of experience is usually taken-for-granted or considered simplistically. Even though a few qualitative studies have focused more directly on experience, most have looked through experience to learning and have not addressed the potentially problematic nature of experience. Having said this, there are a small number of studies which do begin to examine the nature of experience and the connection with learning. Notably, these studies consider the relational nature of experience in the context of time and place. In concert with Selman's (1988) argument, they recognize the character of learning to be social and relational, and more than just an internal process.

It is also somewhat surprising, given the claim that experiential learning involves the whole person, that the body is almost completely overlooked by the experiential learning theorists and only minimally addressed by researchers studying learning experiences. Although Griffin (1987) and Denis & Richter (1987) address intuitive experience, and Griffin (1987), Gray-Snelgrove (1982) and Jarvis (1987a) allude to the body, in general references to bodily experience and the development of bodily knowing are noticeable by their absence. Just as the body is separated from the mind in most of the studies, other notions are also unduly separated. Many of these studies, particularly those underpinning the experiential learning models, separate learning/reflection, learning/experience, and action/reflection. It is notable that these demarcations are not made as sharply in the studies concerning learning in the midst of everyday experience.

Concentrating on the mechanisms or processes of learning, these studies of learning and experience have not always identified specific outcomes of learning. However, when the overall goals of learning are mentioned, autonomy is frequently among them (Merriam 1987), along with greater understanding, personal growth and knowledge of one sort or another. It is to knowledge and the development of expertise that we now turn.

DEVELOPING EXPERTISE

In our common understanding, an expert is someone whose special knowledge or skill causes him or her to be an authority in a particular field or area. Likewise, expertise consists of expert knowledge or opinion. Although it is still unclear just how expertise develops, the close link between experience and becoming expert is reflected in the words' etymological connection with 'experiment'. Inherent in both experience and expertise is the active testing, deployment and development of knowledge and skill.

At the centre of much of the current research on expertise is the concern about how people develop and use knowledge and skill. Most studies aim to discover how people think and make decisions in simulated or real conditions. The researchers' underlying views of knowledge, skill, and practice greatly influence how the studies depict expertise and its development. Thus, if we are to examine everyday experience in nursing practice and its contribution to the development of nursing expertise, it is important to consider the nature of knowledge and skill in professional practice.

Knowledge in everyday experience

Questions about the nature of knowledge in human experience have been the subject of continuous philosophical debate. It is beyond the scope of this study to review this complex and wide-ranging discussion. Rather, in this discussion I intend to distinguish conceptions of knowledge which underly current research on expertise in nursing practice and to explore some of the issues which surround the connection between knowledge and practice.

Within the discussion about the nature of knowledge, a number of distinctions have arisen: distinctions between commonsense knowledge and specialized knowledge, generalized and particular knowledge, and theoretical and practical knowledge. This last distinction, between theoretical and practical knowledge, or knowing-that and knowing-how (Ryle 1949), is a useful way of considering theory and its connection to practice. Freidson (1986) provides a helpful elaboration of formal knowledge in professional action. He contends that formal knowledge is higher knowledge which remains separated from 'both common, everyday knowledge and non-formal specialized knowledge' (p 3). It is formalized into theories and other abstractions which are designed to provide systematic, reasoned explanation and to justify the facts and activities believed to constitute the world. Usually the subject of research and teaching, formal knowledge is characterized by rationalization: the pervasive use of reason and rational action. According to Freidson, experts are commonly considered to be the 'carriers' of formal knowledge. This view is also held in nursing (cf. Christman 1985). The nursing literature is replete with distinctions of formal knowledge which are to be applied to practice in order to improve the care of patients.

In a profession, the way in which knowledge is conceptualized, described and transmitted, illustrates which types of knowledge have most value and what it means to know (Carper 1978). In common with other professions (Freidson 1986, Clark 1991), what counts as nursing knowledge, with very few exceptions, is theoretical or formal knowledge (Beckstrand 1978, Carper 1978, Visintainer 1986, Meleis 1991). Non-formal ways of knowing are frequently overlooked or diminished in importance in the push to establish nursing's scientific footing. A good illustration of this lies in Carper's (1978) discussion of ways of knowing in nursing.

Through her analysis of the conceptual and syntactical structure of nursing knowledge, Carper proposes four patterns of knowing:

1. Empirics — the science of nursing.
2. Aesthetics — the art of nursing.
3. Personal knowledge.
4. Ethics — moral knowledge.

She contends that the greatest emphasis in nursing is on the science of nursing; the others constitute the 'art' of nursing. However, as she describes them, aesthetics and ethics become various forms of theoretical knowledge: they can be abstracted, objectively described and shared. Personal knowledge is described narrowly; Carper contends that it cannot be shared because it is highly personal, subjective and idiosyncratic. Although Carper makes a case for broadening the consideration of what constitutes 'valid and reliable' knowledge in nursing, she maintains a dichotomy between objective and subjective knowledge and reinforces the superior value of formal knowledge.

Following Heidegger (1962), Polanyi ([1958] 1962), Kuhn (1970) and Dreyfus (1980), Benner (1983, 1984, Benner & Wrubel 1989) argues for making a distinction between theoretical knowledge and practical knowledge which does not follow these objective/subjective lines. She proposes a distinction between knowing which is embedded within a particular situation and knowing which is formal and abstract. Her view of practical knowledge and the connection between theory and practice will be discussed shortly. However, at present, it is useful to note that for Benner, theoretical knowledge is abstract:

A formal statement of the necessary and sufficient conditions for the occurrence of real situations. Theoretical knowledge is 'knowing that' and includes formal statements about interactional and causal relationships between events. (Benner 1984 p 298)

This definition is not unlike Meleis' description of nursing theory which shows the influence of, amongst others, Dickoff & James (1975). To Meleis, nursing theory is:

... an articulated and communicated conceptualization of invented or discovered reality (central phenomena and relationships) in or pertaining to nursing for the purpose of describing, explaining, predicting, or prescribing nursing care. (Meleis 1991 p 17)

Both definitions illustrate the fact that theoretical knowledge is abstract, definite, specifically related and readily communicated. It ranges from systematic knowledge that names and categorizes, to knowledge which tells what activities are necessary to reach a nursing goal. Even though it is commonly held that 'theory begins and ends in practice' (Dickoff & James 1975, McFarlane 1977), the nature of the connection between theoretical knowledge and practice remains an open question. It is to this connection that we now turn.

The theory-practice connection

It has been variously suggested that theoretical knowledge provides the 'basis' of nursing practice (e.g. Rogers 1970), that theory 'guides' the nurse in action (e.g. Jacox 1974) or that the nurse 'applies' theory in practice (e.g. Johnson 1968). Despite these contentions, empirical evidence about how nurses actually use or apply theoretical knowledge in their ongoing, everyday practice is scarce in the nursing literature. Indeed, there is evidence from research in other fields about how practitioners use knowledge (Eraut 1985, Clark 1991) that the notion of the 'application' of theoretical knowledge may be a mistaken one. This is not to say that theoretical knowledge is unimportant, nor to underestimate its positive influence on practice. Indeed, the introduction of the 'nursing process' is a case in point (UK DHSS 1986). It also cannot be forgotten that the formal knowledge which underpins organizational and documentary practices has a considerable influence on nursing practice, much of it positive. (cf. Campbell 1984, Gordon 1986, Campbell & Jackson 1992). Notwithstanding the influence of formal knowledge on the organization, and thus on practitioners, the process through which individual practitioners incorporate formal knowledge into their ongoing practices is not clearly understood (Freidson 1986) and merits closer scrutiny.

Practising from theory

One view of the knowledge-practice connection is that nurses (and other practitioners) practise from a theory, or set of theories. This may be viewed in at least two ways. One perspective is that the nurse practises from broad, normative knowledge, for instance a model, view or perspective of nursing (e.g. Field 1983, Kitson 1986). For example, Adam (1987) contends that this 'theoretical perspective', which can be likened to a precursor to theory, determines the nurse's focus of attention and comes from a conceptual model or from outside nursing. Kitson (1986) has linked the presence of such a perspective, on the part of ward sisters, to the quality of care provided in the ward. Others (e.g. Field 1980) emphasize that formal knowledge forms only a part of the nurse's 'horizon' whereby the nurse understands and interprets specific situations, and determines the goals for care.

In the not dissimilar fields of community voluntary action and social work, Clark (1991) underlines this position. He found that rather than working from a model for practice, practitioners were guided by 'a set of action beliefs and dispositions which draws variously on the whole spectrum of the individual's knowledge, values, biography and experience' (p 155). Theoretical knowledge was only a minor part of this set. If the formal knowledge, or theoretical perspective accounts for only a part of how a nurse practices, then the link between theoretical knowledge and practice remains difficult to discern. Considering the connection between practice and a more specific notion of theory may be more productive.

Practice as applying theory

A much narrower notion of theory underpins the second view of the relationship in which theory guides practice. One manifestation is situation-producing theory (Dickoff & James 1975), which prescribes nursing practice from knowledge arising from predictive, causal, correlational and descriptive theories. In practice, the nurses would work from the prescriptive, normative theory, applying it as a template to their practice. Any mismatch between practice and theory would constitute a testing of the theory and thus the theory could be revised and new formal knowledge created. Although knowledge would not stand completely apart from action and would be generated from action, the knowledge thus developed would be a refinement of formal knowledge. Grypdonck (1980, 1987) has demonstrated the use of situation-producing theory in implementing the nursing process and notes how it helps the nurses to improve their care by strengthening the cognitive aspects of it. The theory of nursing process has been refined, for instance, through a reassessment of the need for written communication (Grypdonck 1987).

Theory as a pointer

A less restrictive notion of the connection between theory and practice is provided by Benner (1984, Benner & Wrubel 1989). She suggests that theory is useful for pointing to an area of practice, and for guiding the novice.

Theory is crucial to forming the right questions to ask in a clinical situation; theory tells the practitioner where to look for problems and how to anticipate care needs. (Benner 1984 p 178)

Benner's view is that although theory may be useful to practitioners, it is always secondary to practice, and it is derived from practice. Nevertheless, the notion of theory guiding practice is problematic in an occupation such as nursing where there are more uncharted areas of practice than there are areas in which formal knowledge has been sufficiently developed to act as a guide. Nurses frequently encounter new situations in practice without the benefit of specific theory. Benner recognizes that there are many situations which may be 'beyond' theory, and reiterates that there is more to any situation than a theory predicts. She further suggests that nurses use theory differently as they develop expertise. This point will shortly be more fully explored.

Using and transforming formal knowledge

Freidson (1986), in discussing the institutionalization of formal knowledge, adds an important dimension to this discussion. He suggests that the formal knowledge of a profession advanced by academics and researchers is 'used selectively and transformed in the course of its use' by administrators and practitioners (p 217). In the every workday situation, formal knowledge is '... employed inconsistently and informally. In each case a different transformation of formal knowledge into "working knowledge" (Kennedy 1983) takes place' (Freidson 1986 p 227).

Working knowledge is considered by Kennedy (1983) to be an organized body of knowledge which is used spontaneously and routinely in the context of work.

Theories-in-use

Schön (1983, 1987) challenges what he calls the prevailing view of professional action, 'technical rationality' and offers an alternative way of linking theory and practice. Despite Schön's attention to intuition and practical knowledge, it would seem that his underlying view of the world is essentially the same as the prevailing view. However, because some of his notions are particularly useful, it is important to consider his work here. As mentioned earlier, Argyris & Schön (1974) distinguish two levels at which theories of interpersonal behaviour operate: espoused theories which people use to explain or justify their behaviour, and theories-in-use, which are implicit in patterns of spontaneous behaviour with others. Theories-in-use are a kind of knowing-in-action and are usually tacit. However, theories-in-use can be constructed (or reconstructed) through '... reflecting on the directly observable data of ... actual interpersonal practice ...' (Schön 1987 p 256). Argyris & Schön's 'reflective practicum' through which they teach counselling and consulting skills is aimed at facilitating this process.

Schön (1983, 1987) cogently argues against the normative view of professional practice, in which formal knowledge takes precedence over knowing how and know-how takes the form of science-based technique. Schön counters this view with a proposal for professional practice in which practitioners operate openly, with congruency between their espoused theories and their theories-in-use. In this revised view of practice, one's theories-in-use are the subject of reflection, a kind of reflecting-in-action which 'accounts for artistry in situations of uniqueness and uncertainty' (Schön 1983 p 165).

In arguing for the interconnection of knowing and doing in a new epistemology of practice, Schön (1983) considers knowing-in-action to be tacit knowledge, implicit in patterns of intelligent, practical action. '[We] behave according to rules and procedures that we cannot usually describe and of which we are often unaware' (pp 53–54). Schön's view that knowing-in-action is based upon rules and procedures fits with his understanding that practitioners are actors in a behavioural world, operating from theories-in-use which, potentially, can be articulated.

The second and complementary path in Schön's argument is reflection-in-action, the holding of 'reflective conversations' with one's own practice. He suggests that important to this process are the constants in an occupation: the media, language and normal repertoires that practitioners use to describe reality and conduct experiments; the appreciative systems with which they frame and set problems; the overarching theory by which they make sense of phenomena and the role frames within which they set their tasks. 'They give the practitioner the relatively solid references from which, in reflection-in-action, he can allow his theories and frames to come apart' (p 270). Whilst the notion of reflection-in-action is a helpful one, Schön's use of it suggests that the process of reflecting-in-action is one of testing and revising one's theories-in-use.

Although his focus has changed slightly, Schön's recent works expand and deepen the theme begun in his earlier work with Argyris: that individuals use (implicit) theories-in-action, that theories can be constructed from an individual's knowing-in-practice, and that the individual's implicit knowledge can and should become explicit for the improvement of practice. This would happen through reflective conversation or reflection-in-action. However, despite the recognition of the tacit realm, and the importance of knowing-in-action, Schön maintains a view of the primacy of theory and a dichotomous view of the person and the world.

The interplay of knowledge and practice

The notion of using knowledge permeates the literature on the theory-practice connection. It provides, perhaps, the unifying tie. In the conventional position, the practitioner is viewed as an independent actor with a bag-full of knowledge to be applied or used selectively in specific situations. Theoretical knowledge is foremost: it is applied to practice by a thinking, knowing person (subject) in a separate, object world. A move away from the conventional view is made partially by Schön, but more so by Freidson and Benner. Benner perhaps goes furthest, in following Heidegger's turn to the primacy of practice, in which the subject/object dichotomy is eliminated.

It is timely to review some of the questions which remain about the nature of the connection between theory and practice. These questions are of particular interest when considering the interplay between knowledge and practice in everyday, moment-by-moment nursing practice. As theory is necessarily reductionistic, abstract and atemporal, how does it fit into the rich, ever-changing world of ongoing experience and practice? If formal knowledge changes in a context, as Freidson suggests, what happens in the transformation? Without a separation of subject and object can 'theories-in-use' be recognized in practice? What would influence the 'fit' of a theory, albeit a grounded theory, in a context outwith the one in which it was generated? All of these questions suggest that the nature of the relationship between theory and practice is not only influenced by a view of theory but also by the view of the nature of practice and practical knowledge.

Practical knowledge

Practical knowledge, know-how in everyday situations, is part and parcel of ongoing, everyday action. Practical knowledge is understandably overlooked by writers on theory in nursing (cf. Dickoff & James 1968, Jacox 1974, Meleis 1991), because it is often tacit (Polanyi [1958]1962), situation specific, taken-for-granted and part of our social background practices (Dreyfus 1980). In the currency of an occupation's 'academic professionalizers' (Melia 1987), practical knowledge has a much lower value than formal knowledge. Knowledge which is practical, intuitive and experiential has lost ground in nursing to knowledge that is more scientific and theoretical. There are a number of possibilities why this might be so. Gordon (1986) suggests one:

Practical knowledge appears to symbolize a real and perceived nursing past characterized by subordination to physicians (as physicians' handmaidens), guided by obedience, habit, tradition or women's intuition. It recalls a time when nurses knew only how and not why. (p 959)

Nursing is not the only occupation which has devalued practical knowledge. The recent efforts to describe the 'personal practical knowledge' of classroom teachers is an attempt to redress the imbalance in education (Clandinin & Connelly 1987, Clandinin 1989). In nursing, Benner (1984) provided the first extensive, systematic exploration of practical knowledge in clinical practice through the AMICAE Project. This study of over 1200 nurses in the San Francisco area was originally designed to develop methods of evaluation for participating nursing schools and hospitals. The nurses provided critical incidents (Flanagan 1954) of their nursing practice. Additionally, 21 pairs of novice nurses and their experienced nurse preceptors were studied to ascertain the differences in clinical performance and appraisal of nursing care situations in which they were both involved. Further interviews and/or participant observations were conducted with 51 experienced clinical nurses, 11 newly graduated nurses and five senior nursing students to delineate and describe characteristics of nursing performance at different stages of skill acquisition. The data were analysed using an interpretative approach rooted in the work of Heidegger (1962), Rabinow & Sullivan (1979) and Taylor (1971). Arising from the data were areas of practical knowledge and domains of nursing practice, which will be addressed later.

Significantly, Benner's analysis does not separate subject/object or knowledge/practice. Practical knowledge, or 'knowing how', according to Benner (1984), is the knowledge derived from experience, from the day-to-day business of caring for patients. Practical knowledge is embodied: it is the skilled know-how of the practitioner who has 'knowledge in his/her fingertips', and comes from involved practical activity. It is everyday, ready-to-hand engagement with the world (Heidegger 1962). Practical knowledge is tacit or ineffable — that is, known, but not always capable of being explicitly described. Indeed, 'we can know more than we can tell' (Polanyi 1966). Practical knowledge is personal, but it is not necessarily subjective, private or idiosyncratic. It can be described and shared.

Central to practical knowledge is perception and a perceptual grasp (Merleau-Ponty 1962). For instance, we recognize a face directly: we do not analyze and add the various parts. Pattern recognition, the recognition of similarities and differences, is an essential part of 'normal' human life (Sacks 1985). The ways in which we recognize and understand patterns stem from our engagement in social background practices. These accrue through experience, over time. The patterns include understanding such things as the particulars of social space in different situations and the meanings of the phrasing, timing, tempo or intonation of words in particular contexts. An example of the nuances of practical knowledge which cannot be captured as acontextual, theoretical knowledge was my inability, after nearly four years in Scotland, to be absolutely sure when someone was saying 'no' in some social situations. To my Canadian ear, the meaning of indirect acceptance or refusal was not always clear. I fully understood it in some contexts but not in others. The meaning of particular situations plays an essential role in determining what counts in that situation and 'it is precisely this contextual meaning that theory must ignore' (Dreyfus 1983 p 11). Not searching for theory, Benner identified areas of practical knowledge.

Areas of practical knowledge

In her 1984 work, Benner identified six areas of practical knowledge from the critical incidents, interviews and observations of practice situations:

1. graded qualitative distinctions
2. common meanings
3. assumptions, expectations and sets
4. paradigm cases and personal knowledge
5. maxims
6. unplanned practices.

These areas provide a sense of the range of know-how, and illustrate how knowledge is embedded in clinical practice.

Graded qualitative distinctions: Graded qualitative distinctions are those fine differences in the perceptual grasp of a situation that experienced nurses have learned to make. This perceptual grasp is situation-specific and context-dependent. For example, subtle changes in a patient's wound drainage take on meaning only in light of the patient's current situation and history. Polanyi ([1958]1962) calls this subtle, perceptual grading, 'connoisseurship', and notes that it must be learned through experience. It persists 'because it has not been possible to replace it by a measurable grading' (p 55).

Common meanings: Common meanings are developed by nurses working in similar areas with common issues about health and illness. They evolve over time and are shared among nurses. They are part of a tradition and are embedded in the language used by nurses in particular areas. Using the approach advocated by Benner to examine clinical knowledge, Olsen (1985) and Crabtree & Jorgenson (1986) have identified how death has common meanings for nurses within a specific specialty but that the meanings differ between specialties.

Death in oncology nursing is treated as a life event, and the role assumed by these nurses is one of making this experience as 'good' as possible ... Death ... has been transformed in the ICU [Intensive Care Unit]; it has become a symptom, a harbinger of danger that demands immediate response and treatment. (Crabtree & Jorgenson 1986 pp 187–189)

Assumptions, expectations and sets: Assumptions, expectations and sets imbue the contextual, narrative accounts of nursing practice. For example, assumptions and expectations about patient progress underly nursing actions, assessments and interventions. Assumptions and expectations may be evident to the outside observer and can sometimes be verbalized. Sets, 'a predisposition to act in certain ways in particular situations' (Benner 1984 p 7), determine how a nurse perceives and describes a situation. They are similar to Clark's (1991) 'set of action beliefs and dispositions'. Sets can never be made completely explicit while remaining unchanged. The act of uncovering them, bringing them to awareness, changes their function.

Paradigm cases: Through experience, nurses store and retain vivid memories of significant events. Benner (1984) coined them 'paradigm cases', following Kuhn (1970). Paradigm cases are defined by Benner (1984) as:

A clinical episode that alters one's way of understanding and perceiving future clinical situations. These cases stand out in the clinician's mind; they are reference points in their current clinical practice. (p 296)

Benner contends that past situations stand out because they have changed the nurse's pre-conceptions and prior understandings — his or her personal knowledge. The transaction between this personal knowledge and the clinical situation determines the actions and decisions that the nurse takes. Benner's notion of paradigm case is directly linked to her understanding of experience, which 'results when preconceived notions and expectations are challenged, refined, or discon-firmed by the actual situation' (p 3). We will be returning to the issue of the nature of experience and its link to the nature and role of paradigm cases in Chapter 4 and Chapter 8.

Maxims and unplanned practices: Benner describes

maxims (Polanyi [1958]1962) as cryptic descriptions of skilled performance that can be understood by one who has enough skill and practical know-how to recognize the implications of the instructions. *Unplanned practices* occur when a nurse 'inherits' a new or risky procedure because the nurse is the one present at the patient's bedside when it needs to be done. The nurse 'improvises' and learns to perform this new skill.

Whilst these 'areas of practical knowledge' are useful for becoming attuned to different ways in which practical knowledge can be exhibited and used, their conceptual inconsistency limits their use as a framework through which to explore the everyday experience in nursing practice. In her later work, Benner (1991, 1994) has continued to explore common meanings, paradigm cases and qualitative distinctions in nursing practice. However, the explicit distinction of these areas of practical knowledge has remained in the background; the substance of practical knowledge they reveal has been in the foreground.

Researchers who have explored practical knowledge in nursing using a similar approach to Benner's (e.g. Olsen 1985, Fenton 1985, Crabtree & Jorgenson 1986, Brykczynski 1989, Diekelmann 1989, 1992, 1993, Horvath et al 1994) have extensively used the paradigm case as a unit of analysis. The researchers acknowledge that all of the nuances and the temporal nature of a situation can never be communicated. They contend however, that the richness of practical knowledge can be conveyed through themes, examples, and maxims, and in person, by showing, touching or pointing out smells.

Unlike approaches in which analytical frameworks are laid over descriptions of nursing practice like a template, hermeneutic interpretation of practical knowledge enables the complexity of knowledge to become visible. When she used a traditional content analysis approach, Elster (1987) admitted to having great difficulty in identifying Carper's (1978) ways of knowing in nursing practice. Elster attempted to identify Carper's framework from an analysis of interviews with 14 'excellent' nurses about their nursing practice. She found that when the

nurses' words were taken out of context, their semantic variation was so great that classification was valueless. The interpretation of practical knowledge from the perspective of hermeneutic phenomenology averts this problem of semantic variation, because context and the concomitant meaning are retained during analysis and interpretation, and the knowledge embedded in practice is revealed.

In the section on learning and experience, it was shown that experience is often taken for granted in the quest to examine learning. In much of the research on experiential learning, processes which enhance reflection on theoretical knowledge are emphasized and knowledge embedded in everyday practice and experience is overlooked. The separation of theory and practice parallels the separation of learning and experience. Yet experience is critical in the development of expertise. By examining some of the research on expertise, the nature and role of experience in the development of expertise can be considered further.

Approaches to expertise

The terms 'novice' and 'expert' were first used by the cognitive science and artificial intelligence disciplines, and have been incorporated into the study of performance in other fields (Bereiter & Scardamalia 1986). Studying the contrast between the knowledge and skills of experts and novices has yielded insights into thinking and decision-making skills. Glaser (1987) suggests that studies in cognitive psychology have found expert performance to be characterized by 'rapid access to an organized body of conceptual and procedural knowledge'. The process of decision-making, the nature of this 'rapid access' and the knowledge which is used have been the focus of studies of clinical judgement in nursing (Tanner 1983, Tanner 1987, LeBreck 1989). Most studies have stemmed from the conventional approaches of statistical modelling and information processing (Tanner 1983, LeBreck 1989). However, the use of simulation and analytic procedures in these studies has been found to be of limited help in describing clinical judgement in natural settings because practical knowledge and the influence of the context have been overlooked (Tanner 1989).

In a marked departure from conventional approaches, Benner (1984) used the 'Dreyfus Model of Skill Acquisition' (Dreyfus 1982, Dreyfus & Dreyfus 1986) in the AMICAE study to explore the differences in practice between experienced and less experienced nurses. The Dreyfus Model was first developed during studies of airline pilots and chess players and, before Benner's study, had been extended to the study of automobile drivers and adult learners of a second language. It is unique in its emphasis on the situation-specific nature of the knowledge inherent in expertise (practical knowledge) and the importance of experience in the development of that knowledge. Although the Dreyfus Model presents a unique approach to understanding expertise, it is not alone in recognizing the value of practical knowledge. Other researchers (e.g. Pyles & Stern 1983, Isenberg 1984, Scribner 1986, Grant & Marsden 1988) have also begun to examine the contribution of practical knowledge to expertise and its development through experience.

The Dreyfus Model proposes that, in acquiring expertise in a particular field, people pass through five stages of qualitatively different perceptions of coming to the task and/or modes of decision-making. Expertise is developed along three dimensions: there is a shift from relying on abstract principles to perceive and interpret problems to using past experience as a base for judgement; there is a change from understanding parts of a situation and building a whole picture, to an immediate grasp of the whole situation; there is a shift from being detached and 'outside' the situation to a stance of being involved in the situation. The Model is sufficiently important to merit a fuller explication of the five levels: novice, advanced beginner, competent, proficient, and expert.

1. **Level 1. Novice:** At this stage, the individual has no background knowledge of the situation. The novice performer uses context-free rules to guide action. The rules are principle-based and

theoretical, and concern the objective attributes of a situation.

2. **Level 2. Advanced beginner:** At this stage the nurse has experienced enough real situations to note recurring meaningful components of the situation. The nurse operates with general guidelines and needs help to set priorities. The advanced beginner cannot sort out what is important in complex situations and needs help in aspect recognition.

3. **Level 3. Competent:** The nurse at this stage typically plans his or her care deliberately and consciously. These plans determine which aspects of the situation are most important. He or she is said to be able to 'see the whole picture' or 'be organized'. There is a sense of mastery, of being able to manage or cope with many of the contingencies of clinical practice. The speed and flexibility of the proficient nurse is not yet there.

4. **Level 4. Proficient:** Unlike the competent nurse who still perceives the situation in terms of its aspects, the proficient performer perceives situations as wholes. The proficient performer has an intuitive grasp of the whole based upon deep involvement and recognition of similar patterns. The nurse has experienced many such situations before. Setting priorities and making decisions is less laboured as the nurse recognizes which of the many aspects are most salient. He or she considers fewer options and is able to hone in on the most important region of a problem. Although there is intuitive, holistic recognition of the situation, the proficient nurse still needs to make decisions with detached calculation and reliance on a learned principle (maxim).

5. **Level 5. Expert:** The nurse operating at this level no longer needs to rely on operating principles (rules, guidelines or maxims) to link recognition of the whole situation to appropriate action. The expert has an enormous reserve of experienced situations to draw upon. He or she uses them to assess a problem, accurately hone in on where an intervention should take place, and act. Not only is the perception of the situation intuitive, but so also are the decisions and action.

Dreyfus & Dreyfus and Benner emphasize that

these are stages of performance, not descriptors of people and that the stage of performance can change as the situation changes. However, in their writings, both Dreyfus & Dreyfus (1986) and Benner (1984, Benner et al 1992) persist in naming people 'experts' and 'novices'.

At the core of the Dreyfus Model is the movement from dependence upon theoretical knowledge to practical knowledge, from rational action to intuitive understanding. Dreyfus & Dreyfus propose that intuition is a central component of practical knowledge and is a key to expert clinical judgement. Intuition is defined as 'understanding without a rationale'. It is not, however, an alternate form of cognitive skill (Rew 1986) or an unreliable, commonsense source of knowledge (Fishbein 1985). Dreyfus & Dreyfus note that intuitive judgement is characterized by six key aspects: pattern recognition, similarity recognition, commonsense understanding, a sense of salience, skilled know-how and deliberative rationality. Benner & Tanner (1987) have identified these aspects in their pilot study of expert clinical nursing decision-making. They also form the core of the Dreyfus Model's proficient and expert levels. Although action is discussed, it is often superseded by issues of decision-making. Until recently (Benner et al 1992) there has been little explicit discussion by Dreyfus & Dreyfus or Benner of the process of developing physical abilities, or of the suitability of action to the situation.

A key issue which the Dreyfus Model does not sufficiently address concerns how people move from one level of skill to another. It is suggested that this movement happens by the 'accumulation' of an immense 'library of distinguishable situations' which is built up on the basis of experience (Dreyfus & Dreyfus 1986 p 32). They further suggest that people make a qualitative 'jump' between stages, rather than progress in a linear fashion. Benner (1991) describes narratives of learning that depict practical knowledge and ethical comportment and assist nurses to develop expertise. The nature of experience and the process of

accumulation, however, remain underexplored. Also needing further examination is the interplay between theoretical knowledge and practical knowledge during reflection.

The contribution of reflection

As we have seen, reflection is central to the experiential learning models and to Schön's (1983) epistemology of professional practice. The actual process of reflection is variously described in the models, but commonly reflection is deliberate, conscious, analytical and occurs outwith the flow of action. Schön contends, however, that some practitioners integrate reflection into a smooth flow of action as reflection-in-action. Unfortunately, Schön's notion of action in practice is confusing as it encompasses both immediate and lengthy time frames. Schön suggests that reflection-in-action may occur over a number of minutes, or a number of months.

The process of reflection enters the Dreyfus Model in several ways. Up to the level of expert performance, reflection and planning is prior to and part of action. However, at the expert stage, reflection is retrospective: the expert acts intuitively, then critically reflects on those intuitions. Dreyfus & Dreyfus note how destructive it can be to fluid performance in familiar circumstances when the expert reflects prior to action. However, 'when time permits and outcomes are crucial, an expert will deliberate before acting' (pp 31–32).

Dreyfus & Dreyfus are particular about what type of reflection is most helpful in developing practical expertise. They contend that the mode of reflection changes with experience from 'calculative rationality' (objective, distanced and analytical) to 'deliberative rationality' (involved, synthetic and perspective changing) (Benner & Tanner 1987). Deliberative rationality, a form of practical reasoning, comprises:

1. Contemplating the differences in the situation to account for the differences.
2. Focusing on the overall plan and noticing

issues arising as the plan is played out.

3. Experiencing a change of perspective on the situation, so that new issues arise.

4. Considering the relevance and adequacy of past situations which seem to underly a current situation (Dreyfus & Dreyfus 1986).

At the higher levels of skilled performance deliberative rationality or practical reflection is used to free oneself from 'stuckness' (Pirsig 1974). It could be said that when engaged in practical reflection, the practitioner dwells within the situation in such a way that there is an openness to what may not have been previously seen or understood. Dreyfus & Dreyfus talk about the changes in the nature of reflection with each of the skill stages. In their discussion, however, they do not elaborate on just how practitioners can move from one stage to another.

Reflection in some form seems to be an essential feature of the development of expertise. If reflection is as conscious and rational as some theorists lead us to believe (e.g. Mezirow 1990), we should be able to report it. However, there is some evidence to the contrary. In some studies of learning, people have been unable to give sensible reports of their learning from introspection (cf. Nisbett & Wilson 1977). In addition, learning that occurs without conscious thought has been found to be inaccessible through verbal reports (cf. Bellezza 1986). Dreyfus & Dreyfus (1986) suggest that for learning to occur a part of the mind must remain aloof in order to monitor the situation. On rare occasions, however, during exceptional, fluid practice, monitoring ceases. The question remains about whether learning is occurring during such periods of fluid practice, and indeed what is the nature of experience during those times. It would appear, that like experience, reflection is something of a familiar but poorly understood entity. We can speculate about what goes on within reflection, but cannot entirely understand it. This is particularly the case with reflection in everyday practice. If, like Dreyfus & Dreyfus, we take the view that the conventional dichotomies between subject/object,

action/reflection are misplaced when considering everyday practice and the development of expertise, then we cannot help but find the nature of the relationship between practice, practical knowledge and theoretical understanding to be problematic.

Summary

Conventional approaches to the question of expertise have come from a perspective which accords primary value to formal or theoretical knowledge (knowing-that). In this perspective, theoretical knowledge is commonly used as an explicit guide to practice. Overlooked in this perspective is practical knowledge, or knowing-how. Almost singularly amongst the approaches to decision-making the Dreyfus Model of Skill Acquisition recognizes the contextual nature of expertise and the importance of practical know-how. The Model is also unique in its attention to the role of experience in developing expertise. Although Benner's research with the Dreyfus Model provides a good opening to the understanding of expertise in nursing practice, some problems and unexamined areas remain. Notably, the model focuses on the decision-making aspect of performance to the exclusion of other areas of performance and their development. Experience is considered to be relatively non-problematic and the nature of learning itself is not fully explored.

CONCLUDING REMARKS

In this chapter, I have examined two bodies of knowledge: research on learning and experience and research on knowledge and the development of expertise. We have seen that experience, though much discussed, is little examined, and when it is examined, it is treated by most theorists in adult learning as a non-problematic, static entity. Most of the studies and the models developed from them maintain a central focus on learning. Those studies which take a phenomenological approach, particularly those which concentrate on natural or incidental learning experiences, consider experience more closely and reveal more of its complexity.

The conventional view of the link between theory and practice, in which theory precedes and is applied in practice, was explored and found to be wanting. An alternative approach to the link between theory and practice and the development of expertise, as exemplified by the Dreyfus Model of Skill Acquisition, was explored. This approach, which suggests that practical knowledge is primary, was shown to hold promise for illuminating the contribution of everyday experience to the development of nursing expertise. Of particular note was its concern with considering expertise in context. It is to nursing practice, the context of nursing expertise and experience, that we now turn.

3

Nursing practice: the context of nursing experience

INTRODUCTION

Nurses' everyday practice provides the context for nursing experience and for the development of nursing expertise. The focus of this chapter is on how nursing practice, particularly the practice of ward sisters, is depicted in the research literature. Special attention is paid to those studies which attend to nurses' experience in practice. Before turning to the research literature, however, it is useful to recall why we focus on the ward sister. In Chapter 1 we saw how most of the nurses identified by the senior nursing managers as 'excellent, experienced, clinical nurses' were ward sisters.

It is not unusual to identify clinical expertise at the ward sister level, even with the introduction of clinical specialists throughout the system. Despite the increased emphasis on the management aspects of the role, the ward sister (or charge nurse) is generally expected to be '... a role model for ward staff and a repository of clinical expertise' (Lathlean 1987 p 16). This assumption of clinical competence permeates the ward sister literature, which concentrates, for the most part, on the management role, and stemming from this, the teaching role. Paradoxically, the clinical role of first-line nursing managers in general, and of the ward sister in particular, remains little explored (Choppin 1983, Duffield 1991), overlooked and somewhat taken for granted.

The charge nurse/ward sister is considered to be the first management level in the National Health Service (NHS) (UK Ministry of Health 1966, UK Parliament 1979, Abel et al 1986). Like the North American head nurse, unit manager or nurse manager, the ward sister is the level where the clinical and managerial roles meet most sharply. The charge nurse/sister is the key figure in the ward team. He/she is responsible for: overall planning and standards of care; developing ward policies; delegating authority within the nursing team to facilitate work; and assessing patients' needs, setting objectives and monitoring progress (UK Parliament 1972).

Increasingly, the ward sister is assuming responsibility for resource management, staffing and budgeting. The importance and influence of the ward sister in the ward, and the complexity of the role, are recurring themes in research reports and reports emanating from committees, statutory and professional bodies. With continuing organizational changes, the complexity of the role is unlikely to diminish.

Nursing practice itself has been studied from various perspectives: the roles, tasks and activities undertaken by nurses, the process of nursing, the particular problems with which nurses are concerned, and most recently, the domains of nursing practice (McFarlane 1989). This delineation provides a useful organizing framework for the discussion which follows.

NURSING ROLES: TASKS AND ACTIVITIES

Perhaps the first and most enduring approach to the study of nursing practice has been the description and analysis of tasks and activities. One of the first of these studies was the job analysis undertaken for the Working Party on the Recruitment and Training of Nurses (UK Ministry of Health 1947). Stemming from that report was Goddard's (1953) study of the work of nurses in hospitals which became a touchstone for other researchers. Goddard used quantitative work study methods to answer the question, 'What is the proper task of a nurse?'. For the purposes of task analysis, he categorized nursing duties into the following:

1. 'basic' nursing
2. 'technical' nursing
3. administration and organization

4. domestic work
5. miscellaneous.

'Basic' nursing care was originally defined as the care required for the physical comfort of the patient; 'technical' nursing care included the tasks concerned 'with the treatment of the disease from which the patient is suffering' (p 37). These categories, sometimes with modifications, continued to be used over the next three decades by other researchers (cf. Revans 1964, Bendall 1975, Moult et al 1978, Fretwell 1982).

Bendall's research provides a useful illustration. To ascertain the relationship between knowledge and practice, Bendall (1973, 1975) extended Goddard's categories to study the activities of learners in the ward and compared these activities to what the learners said they would do in a given situation. Finding a very considerable discrepancy (73%), Bendall concluded that there was a marked conflict between the ideal and the real. Notwithstanding the potential importance of this difference, it is notable that Bendall did not question the adequacy of task analysis for depicting situational nursing practice.

The limitations of the task analysis approach was readily recognized by Goddard (1953) when he stated, 'Any attempt to analyse this type of work inevitably results in a cold, calculated list of duties and fails to convey the atmosphere in which the duties are performed'. He noted that this approach omits aspects of nursing work, for example, how nurses 'exercise constant vigilance towards the patient's condition' (p 25). However, the benefits of a scientific, 'completely objective approach' were felt to outweigh these limitations.

A study to compare task and patient allocation systems of ward organization identified the complexity of nursing care and the difficulties inherent in measuring nursing activity by means of rigid categories (Moult et al 1978). Writing about this study, Melia (1979) suggested that a sociological approach, based on role analysis, would be more fruitful. She proposed that the complexity of practice would be more readily captured by describing the nurse's role, where she worked and what kind of nursing skills she made use of in her daily work. To do this, more than observational task analysis would be required. Accordingly, other researchers used more than task analysis in their studies of the role of the ward sister. However, with only one exception (Runciman 1983), the researchers chose to focus on only one aspect of the role.

Ward sisters: the management role

The Briggs Report (UK Parliament 1972), among other studies, stressed the importance of ward management to the quality of nursing practice. Consistent with this view, in perhaps the most influential study of ward sisters in the UK, Pembrey (1980) suggested that the exercise of the managerial role by the ward sister was crucial to the provision of individualized nursing care to patients.

Pembrey identified that those sisters who completed a four-stage management cycle in relation to each nurse and each patient ensured the delivery of individualized patient care. The management cycle consisted of: defining work (a nursing round of patients); prescribing work (written and verbal work prescription); delegating authority to work (allocation of work); and exacting accountability for work (accountability reports). An observational work activity analysis was used to examine the ward sisters' role differentiation. The second classification, of the work of the sister in relation to the ward management cycle, was derived from activity analysis as well as from qualitative criteria. Significantly, only nine of the 50 sisters completed all of the steps of the management cycle; a minority of the sisters completed any one of the four activities in the management cycle. The sisters who did complete the management cycle activities were said to manage the care on an individual patient basis. Whilst this study provides substantial insight into management activities, a view of the patient care which was made possible by these activities is not forthcoming. Additionally, Pembrey's study does not indicate that the sisters achieved multiple goals through seemingly mundane tasks, a phenomenon which Runciman (1983) notes is prevalent in ward sister practice. Indeed, an activity analysis framework such as

Pembrey's overlooks the goals which are inherent in nursing interventions (Glass 1983). Further, as Evers (1982a) points out, and Pembrey acknowledges, research such as this takes the ward and the patient for granted.

Education for the role of ward sister reflects this emphasis on the management skills. The Ward Sister Training Project, an experimental alternative to first-line management courses, was highly influenced by Pembrey's research. The 'implicit notion of the scheme was the development of "manager" sisters' (Lathlean & Farnish 1984 p 3). While the programme was intended to emphasize the managerial role, in the evaluation of the project, Lathlean & Farnish acknowledge the important influence of the ward context on the nature of individual sisters' work.

Ward sisters: the teaching role

The majority of studies of the ward sisters' role concentrate on the teaching component of that role, a concern not reflected in studies of North American or Israeli head nurses (cf. Bergman et al 1981, Hodges et al 1987, Dunn & Schilder 1993). It further highlights the different emphasis in the British nursing education system, where until recently, the learners were part of the workforce and their clinical education and supervision the responsibility of the ward sister.

McGhee (1961) and Revans (1964) were among the first to highlight the importance of ward sisters in determining the ward atmosphere and its influence on patient recovery. The influence of the ward atmosphere on student learning was explored by Fretwell (1978, 1982) and Orton (1981). Not surprisingly, the ward sister was found to be the most important person in setting the tone for learning in the ward. The ward sister 'is the person, above all, responsible for the climate of her ward' (Orton 1981).

Fretwell's (1978, 1982) study attempted to describe and analyse the teaching/learning situations in hospital wards, and to identify the characteristics of a 'good' ward learning environment. Activity analysis was again a central part of the research method. In the first stage of a two-stage project, 327 students rated wards as good or less good. From these ratings, Fretwell constructed characteristics of an 'ideal' ward learning environment. On the ideal ward, sisters and staff nurses:

- Show an interest in the learner when he/she starts on the ward
- Ensure good learner/staff relationships
- Are approachable and available, pleasant yet strict
- Promote good staff/patient relationships and quality of care
- Give support and help to learners
- Invite questions and give answers
- Work as a team.

For the second stage, Fretwell created three high/low pairs of wards from the student ratings. Nursing activities of students were sampled and analysed using categories modelled on systems used by Goddard (1953) and Bendall (1973). Analysis of ward sister activities were developed from a system suggested by Inman (1975). Fretwell found differences in the ward learning environment to be partially related to the sisters' leadership style. These she termed: autocratic, democratic or laissez-faire. To further explain the differences, Fretwell used Bendall's (1973) notion of ward sister orientation: how the sister spent her time and to whom she gave priority. Bendall had identified two orientations: patient orientation and doctor orientation. Fretwell added a third, administration orientation. To measure ward sister orientation, Fretwell turned again to activity analysis, this time 10-minute activity sampling, augmented by qualitative data which was collected during 'key' events.

Fretwell (1982) found that an ideal learning environment is created by the sister and is characterized by teamwork, negotiation and good communication. She suggests that the sister who is democratic, patient-orientated and sees the students as learners rather than workers can create such an environment. 'Those wards in which learners learn a lot are those wards in which sisters make a conscious effort to make teaching a reality' (p 111).

Something of the complexity of the sisters' role comes through in this study, but the contextual nature of both the students' and sisters' practice is missing. The separation of nursing care into activity categories only reflects what tasks are apparently being undertaken. The intention, the goal, the complexity of decision-making and the process of practice are all overlooked in this approach. This separation of activities and tasks runs the very real risk of perpetuating the perception of a hierarchy of skills, with technical skills being more valuable than basic skills (McFarlane 1976).

Students' perceptions provided most of the data for two further studies which examined the ward sisters' role in creating and maintaining an effective learning climate. Orton (1979, 1981) found that the ward learning climate is a 'property of the environment' and exists as a 'psychological reality' for student nurses. On the basis of student responses to two scales which asked about activities and attitudes, Orton was able to discriminate between wards with 'high student orientation' and 'low student orientation'. This discrimination was confirmed by question-naire data from the sisters indicating where they actually did spend their time and where they would prefer to spend their time. Hallmarks of a high student orientation ward were a combination of good patient care, teamwork, consultation and awareness by the ward sister of the needs of her subordinates.

Ogier (1982) sought to develop grounded theory about the leadership style and verbal interactions of ward sisters with nurse learners. She studied the verbal interactions of four ward sisters with nurse learners over the period of a week. The interactions were examined for content and speech form and compared to the results of questionnaires completed by learners about their perceptions of the ward learning climate. Again, a favoured leadership style was identified, one in which the ward sister was approachable, learner-orientated and sufficiently directive for the nature of the work. Seven years later, these findings were confirmed by a smaller replication study (Ogier 1986). While both Orton's and

Ogier's studies cast some light on aspects of the ward sister role and identify positive attributes of the ward sister, little light is shed by these studies on the actual practices of ward sisters.

In a somewhat differently designed study, Marson (1981) sought to isolate those behaviours of ward teachers (nurses, sisters and others) considered by trainee nurses to help them to learn from work experience. Her study was completed in three phases. The first phase included structured interviews with learners and ward sisters to ascertain perceptions of teaching and learning, and to obtain a description of the behavioural characteristics of a 'good ward teacher'. The second phase sought to test the 'good teacher' findings with a larger group of learners. It is notable that learners did not respond to a request to provide critical incidents of effective learning experiences and Marson replaced this technique with a questionnaire. The third phase consisted of structured observations of verbal interactions and observations of nursing activities.

Although Marson replicated many of the research findings of Orton, Ogier and Fretwell more clearly than the others, she identified that 'on the job' teaching is a complex global act. She does not dwell on the notion of role modelling, but notes that the ways in which the nurse (ward sister) acts during her ongoing practice is critically important when it comes to learners' experiences. Again, however, the context and content of nursing practice are not captured by activity analysis and this phenomenon of 'being a nurse in practice' could not be more fully explored. Marson herself recognizes this need and recommends that further research is undertaken to look into what students learn and how the qualities of good ward teachers can be conveyed to others. Robinson & Elkan (1989) note that these recommendations remain as current as they were when Marson wrote them in 1981.

Ward sisters: the clinical role

I have suggested that the ward sisters' clinical role is so central that it is usually taken for granted and remains in the background of most of the studies of ward sisters. When the role is discussed, it is often in terms of setting and ensuring standards for care (e.g. RCN 1981, Lewis 1990). There is little direct examination of the clinical role itself. Part of the lack of attention may stem from different understandings of the clinical role and its importance.

In a study of the attitudes and activities of ward sisters, undertaken as a precursor to a management training programme in one hospital in Wales, Williams (1969) found that senior nurses attached considerable significance to the sisters' management responsibilities. The sisters, however, attached more significance to their clinical responsibilities. More than 25 years later, there continues to be disagreement about the nature and priorities of the ward sister's role. Perhaps one of the reasons that a clear consensus has not yet been reached, is the difficulty in depicting the nature of the clinical role. Williams (1969) describes the sisters' role as having a clinical core: 'a small kernel of purely professional activity', surrounded by layers of activities which are progressively more managerial. While the clinical activity is central, this metaphor may not be particularly apt, as managerial, clinical and teaching activities would not necessarily be 'layered'. Also, the impression given by other studies (Marson 1982, Runciman 1983), is one of integrated activities.

The centrality of the clinical role is implied in suggestions that the ward sister is a role model for nursing staff and learners (e.g. Marson 1981, 1982, Allen 1982). As students, in particular, are learning to give direct care, it can be assumed that the ward sister is modelling clinical care, rather than management or teaching. Another, more likely possibility, sees the sister modelling integrated, complex practice.

It is of interest that one of the clearest statements about the ward sister's clinical role comes from consultants. In the preparatory phase of a ward sister training programme, Allen (1982) asked consultants in participating training wards to describe their expectations of the ward sisters. Amongst the responsibilities attributed by the consultants to the ward sisters were: smooth running of and reasonable quietness in the ward; comfort and well-being of patients; day-to-day management of food, bowels, sedation, analgesia and general activity; communication with patients' relatives concerning patient details; and arranging appropriate access for patients and relatives to consultant and junior medical staff.

This, of course, gives only one, albeit limited, view of the role of the ward sister, but it is notable that it is a clinically-focused view.

A link between the ward sister's conceptual approach and the outcome of care was made in Kitson's (1986, 1991) study of the quality of care on geriatric wards. Once again, activity analysis was the mode of choice for the objective assessment of practice. Unlike other studies, however, the researcher made qualitative judgements about the suitability of the nurses' actions. Nurse-patient interactions were analysed and judged to be therapeutic or non-therapeutic. The therapeutic goal was to achieve optimal self-care and independence. The scores on this set of measures, the Therapeutic Nursing Function (TNF) Matrix, were explained by the ward sisters' TNF Indicator: a self-administered questionnaire designed to identify aspects of organizational ability, knowledge and attitudes towards care. Kitson found that more therapeutic nurse-patient interactions occurred on wards where the ward sister had a patient-centred or therapeutic nursing care outlook. A major drawback of the study, which Kitson recognizes, is that the research tools are in the developmental stage. Norman et al (1994) examined the value of Kitson's TNF Indicator and Therapeutic Nursing Function Matrix. They propose that the discrepancies between Kitson's and their own findings are likely due to changes in the organization of nursing work. What remain to be examined in both studies, however, are the methods of judging quality and the different levels of competency amongst nursing staff. Although the quality of care is addressed, the context of the situations in which the interactions occur remains hidden.

Roles and work

Other studies of the ward sisters' role and the nature of nursing work provide important insights into nursing practice. Redfern (1981) and Runciman (1983) studied the role from the sisters' perspective. Redfern's (1981) study of sisters' job attitudes highlighted the complexity of stresses and conflicts inherent in the role. She found that sisters derived the greatest satisfaction from aspects intrinsic to the work itself, such as helping people. Organizational factors provided the greatest source of dissatisfaction.

In a study which sought depth rather than breadth, Runciman (1983) studied the role from the perspective of problems experienced by nine ward sisters. She undertook an activity analysis over 28 hours of observation with each sister, gathered information about the sisters' self-perception through a semantic differential technique and short interview regarding a shift, and interviewed each at length about problem statements. Unlike other researchers, Runciman highlights the difficulty of identifying and coding units of behaviour because of the complexity of the ward sister actions. Through her examples, Runciman depicts the contextual nature of the sisters' actions and problems and acknowledges the sisters' emphasis on their clinical management role. Runciman's study is particularly helpful for revealing the important and recurring problems of ward sisters' experience in practice, such as interruptions and handling conflicts. The sisters' practice in its ongoing context, however, remains somewhat hidden.

A number of studies using sociological approaches consider the wider context of nursing, including the complex social relationships in a nursing ward. As Evers (1982b) suggests, these studies give insights into the social processes in nursing practice. Strauss et al (1985), for example, describe a number of different dimensions of nursing work and the ways in which it is carried out. Smith (1988, 1992) describes nursing work in terms of emotional labour and links it to the quality of care in a ward. In these studies, the work is separated from the people who do it and the particular ongoing situations in which the nurses practice. For example, Smith talks about nurses 'doing' both emotional labour and technical labour. There is a distinct separation of subject and object in this instrumental approach to practice. Like the sociological studies of experience and learning, these studies quickly move from the starting point of a person's subjective experience to an explanation of the social world. They leave unexplored the relational nature and meaning of ongoing everyday practice.

The studies of nursing roles, for the most part, have concentrated on the delineation and exploration of nursing activities and tasks. A few studies have considered the social context and the social processes of nursing work. Overlooked in these approaches are:

- The ongoing context of practice of which tasks are but a part
- The goals and meaning of practice
- The knowledge and decision-making skills required to care for patients in an appropriate and timely manner
- The interconnected nature of the individual and the social world.

The move to reclaim nursing as a caring profession (McFarlane 1976, Roach 1987, Benner & Wrubel 1989) stems in part from a recognition of the inadequate depiction of nursing practice as simply an amalgam of activities or tasks, separated from the meanings and context within which it happens.

THE NURSING PROCESS

The nursing process, 'a planned, systematic approach to the care of the individual patient' (UK DHSS 1986), has been established as a principle of good nursing (RCN 1980, RCN 1981). Usually, the nursing process is said to consist of four or five stages in a problem-solving process: assessment, diagnosis, planning, implementation and evaluation. The literature on the nursing process is wide ranging because the nursing process has been taken to mean an organizational approach to care, as well as an individual nurse's approach to the care of an individual patient. Included in this range of literature are studies on the knowledge and skills required for the nursing process, implementation of the process, and underlying communication processes and systems.

Research on implementing the nursing process has included studies on organizational changes, changes in work assignment from task to patient assignment, and changes in documentation. These studies will not be explored here as they emphasize the organization of nursing practice. Greater insight into the practice of individual nurses is afforded by research on the generic skills and processes deemed necessary to implement the nursing process (UK DHSS 1986). These include interpersonal relations, communication, clinical decision-making, and psychomotor and measurement skills.

As mentioned in an earlier section, a concentration on the process of decision-making, because it is decontextualized, gives only a limited insight into the nature of everyday practice (Tanner 1983). This is also the case for nursing diagnosis (cf. Gordon 1985, Kim 1989) and nurse-patient interaction and communication (cf. MacLeod Clark 1982, Bottorff & Morse 1994). Lelean's (1973) study serves as a good illustration of the potential and limitations inherent in studies of communication, and of their ability to shed light on the complexities of nursing practice.

Lelean attempted to measure the effectiveness of formal communication between ward sisters and nurses regarding patient care. Eight categories of 'nursing care items' were studied: mobility, toilet, period up, washing/bathing, feeding, turning, blood pressure and 4-hourly TPR. The ward sisters' ratings of the patients' needs for these items on a patient dependency form were compared to observed nursing care, to see whether the nurses were doing what the sisters thought they should be doing for the patients. In addition, the ward sisters' instructions were compared to observed nursing care. In the findings, Lelean describes the amount and duration of the communication between the sisters and various groups of staff. Lelean confirms the findings of Revans (1964) and others that the ward sister is 'the *key person* on the ward controlling all communication coming into and going out of the ward as well as that within the ward itself' (Lelean 1973 p 102).

The limitations of gaining a view of ongoing nursing practice through an analysis of a part are exemplified by the difficulty in classifying the sisters' instructions in a reliable manner. This difficulty was such that Lelean was unable to compare the sisters' instructions with the observed nursing care. For example, 'mobilize' had six different meanings and could mean two different things in one day. The consistency between the patient dependency assessments and observed nursing care in certain categories showed that the sisters and staff shared meaning about some instructions. While Lelean's method allows for a range of meanings to be identified and highlights the imprecision of both verbal and written instructions, it precludes an examination of the meaning of the instructions in particular situations.

Such an acontextual treatment of the study of communication patterns is not uncommon (May 1990). While these studies provide valuable insight into specific components of nursing practice, in their search for general, acontextual knowledge, they present a limited view of nursing practice which frequently emphasizes the deficits of that practice.

PROBLEMS AND CONCERNS OF PRACTICE

An increasing number of studies are examining clinical phenomena (Brown et al 1984, Loomis 1985). In these studies, the focus is on problems such as pain (Seers 1987, Closs 1992), the experience of patients recovering from surgery or illness (Webb 1984, Ford 1989) or specific nursing interventions (McHugh et al 1982, Devine 1992). Although these studies of the quality of nursing care are, as McFarlane (1970) suggests, 'intrinsically valuable for the light they throw on nursing practice' (p 11), they provide a better view of the phenomena of concern to nurses than they do of nursing practice itself.

For instance, Seers' (1987) study sought to examine the factors affecting pain, pain relief, anxiety and recovery in patients undergoing elective abdominal surgery. Patients were interviewed preoperatively and 14 times postoperatively. Nurses caring for the patient rated pain and pain relief on a verbal rating scale; recovery was estimated daily and trained nurses were asked for their opinions on postoperative relief. Although this study provided rich data about the control of post-surgical pain and the consistencies and discrepancies between nurses' and patients' ratings, the practices of the nurses were only partially revealed. Missing are the important contextual aspects of the nurses' practice in specific patient situations.

Inman (1975), in her assessment of the studies in the Study of Nursing Care project, notes the need for a more comprehensive study of the situational nature of nursing practices. While the studies (e.g. Hayward 1975) were successful in examining the objective aspects of nursing care situations and the attributes of nurses giving care, they were not as successful in addressing the contextual nature of that care and the effect of its situational nature on the quality of nursing care. Twenty years later, the need identified by Inman still remains for most areas of nursing practice.

Missing from the studies of the problems and concerns of nursing practice is an explicit recognition that nursing practice and the quality of care are affected by the competence of the person giving that care (Benner 1984). This oversight is of particular importance when considering the British nursing studies. In almost all of the studies done before the 1990s, much, if not most of the nursing care, was provided by untrained nursing staff: students, pupils or auxiliaries. The picture presented is the nursing care of inexperienced, not yet fully competent practitioners — an important consideration when the view presented is a general view which highlights what is not there (e.g. MacLeod Clark 1982). Unfortunately, the practice of experienced, accomplished nurses is not generally evident.

NURSING PRACTICES

It was said earlier that Benner (1984, Benner & Wrubel 1989, Benner et al 1992) takes a marked departure from previous ways of studying nursing practice. Notably, Benner stresses the importance of recognizing that nursing practice happens in an ongoing situation; that the apparently intuitive, taken-for-granted practices have embedded in them sophisticated knowledge and skills. These knowledge and skills, this practical know-how, is formed and reformed in the ongoing situation. Therefore nursing practices must be studied in their ongoing situation.

In the discussion thus far, a distinction has been made between nursing care and nursing practice. Nursing care refers to specific actions or complexes of actions which nurses perform, while nursing practice concerns the exercise of nursing care. Nursing care is the 'what'; nursing practice combines the 'what' with the 'why', the 'how', the 'when' and the 'where'. Using an interpretative strategy which focuses on meanings as a way of organizing and describing practice, Benner attempts to depict the process, content and context of nursing practice. The context of practice includes 'the timing, meanings, and intentions of the particular situation' (Benner 1982 p 306).

In the AMICAE Project which is described in Chapter 2, Benner (1984) inductively identifies 31 nursing competencies. She suggests that these competencies, which are not adequately identified by their labels (e.g. providing comfort and communication through touch), can only be understood by reference to their contextual examples. The competencies are organized into seven domains of nursing practice:

- The helping role
- The teaching/coaching function
- The diagnostic and patient monitoring function
- Effective management of rapidly changing situations
- Administering and monitoring therapeutic interventions and regimens
- Monitoring and ensuring the quality of health care practices
- Organizational and work role competencies.

Others have used Benner's interpretative approach to study nursing practice. Fenton (1984, 1985) studied masters-prepared nurses; Brykczynski (1989), nurse practitioners; Olsen (1985), oncology nurses; Crabtree & Jorgenson (1986), intensive care nurses. Through their interpretation of paradigm cases, Olsen and Crabtree & Jorgenson confirmed the domains of practice and many of the competencies in them. Fenton (1985) and Steele & Fenton (1988) added the domain of 'the consulting role' from their study of clinical nurse specialists. Brykczynski (1989) interviewed and observed 22 nurse practitioners in an ambulatory care setting. She combined two domains (the 'diagnostic and patient monitoring function' and 'administering and monitoring therapeutic interventions'), incorporating them into a new domain for ambulatory care: 'management of patient health/illness status in ambulatory care settings'.

It is apparent from these studies that whilst most domains of practice are common to all areas of nursing, the specific character and emphasis of the domains differ among specialty areas and among nurses in different roles. Notably, the participants in all of these studies, except Brykczynski's, were identified as experts according to the criteria used by Benner (1984 p 15). The nurses had had at least five years of clinical experience, were currently engaged in direct patient care, and were recognized by their peers and others as being highly skilled clinicians. It would be interesting to see whether the domains of practice and competencies would differ among nurses of lesser competence. As they are inductively derived from specific nursing contexts, it could be expected that the domains and competencies would also differ among countries.

Although the description of competencies and domains, with their accompanying examples, depict the context, content and process of nursing practice, Benner's taxonomic framework does not depict the care of groups of patients. This problem is partially addressed in *The Primacy of Caring* (Benner & Wrubel 1989), in which nursing practice is explored in relation to the 'lived experience of human illness and the relationships among health, illness, and disease'. The practices of expert clinical nurses, characterized as caring practices, help patients to cope with the stress of illnesses such as neurological disease, coronary illness and cancer. Only partially explored are the social and organizational contexts in which nurses work. For the most part, the focus remains on the caring practices of individual nurses. Caring practices, as described by Benner & Wrubel, are always understood in a context: they are specific and relational. That is, the practices always stand in relation to the particular nature of the situation; they develop and unfold as the situation unfolds. They both create and are created by the situation itself.

One disadvantage of Benner's approach is that the view of nursing practice is always through the nurse: the research material, the interviews and paradigm cases come from the nurses. The patients' understanding of and actions in the situation are revealed only through the nurses' accounts. It is left to other researchers (e.g. Stainton 1992, Rittman et al 1993, Darbyshire 1994, Wros 1993, 1994) to directly explore the experiences of patients and their families.

Participant observation, which promises a broader perspective, has been used by Benner and others, but seems to play a secondary, confirmatory role. However, it is interesting that in *From novice to expert* some examples, for instance the hazards of immobility, are from participant observation field notes. This pattern

of exemplars is not explained. Benner concedes that the research material is biased towards the dramatic and poignant, at the expense of the mundane, because the research strategy requested 'outstanding clinical situations' (p xxii). Additionally, because the research approach seeks to describe skilled practice, deficits are not examined. That which is present in the narratives and the observational instances is studied; that which is not present receives lesser attention (cf. Fenton 1984, 1985). However, despite these drawbacks, Benner's approach, which concentrates on the particulars of practice in specific contexts, seems to be more successful in depicting the complexity of nursing practice than are previous approaches.

In addition to the studies which have approached nursing practice from the perspective of hermeneutic phenomenology, other researchers have examined nurses' subjective experiences using more traditional phenomenological approaches (Beck 1994). For example, Field (1981) examined nurses' experiences of giving an injection, and Forrest (1989) explored 17 hospital staff nurses' subjective experience of caring. These studies do contribute important insights to the understanding of nursing practice. However, like the studies of the experience of learners which take a traditional phenomenological approach, they still maintain the subjective/ objective dichotomy. In addition, the categories and themes which are developed from the material are somewhat abstract, and the situational and relational nature of nursing practice is not as fully developed as it might be.

In these phenomenological studies, and in those using hermeneutic phenomenology, the nurses' experiences, related in interviews or written in essays or paradigm cases, are treated non-problematically. The researchers are interested in the content of the experiences; on interpreting the 'meanings, situations, practices and bodily experiences' (Benner 1985), or extracting and 'formulating meanings' (Forrest 1989) from the descriptions of lived experiences. In the discussions about method, the forms of the experiences are not examined in depth. Once in textual form, the experiences appear to be treated rather like vessels of feelings and meanings, albeit vessels which hold experiences which have taken place over time. This issue, about the form and nature of experience, will be taken up in the next chapter.

CONCLUDING REMARKS

In summary, nursing practice has a history of being studied from a number of perspectives which fracture its various parts and fail to capture and convey its complex, contextual nature. This is especially so for a role like that of the ward sister. In particular, the clinical component of the ward sister role, while central, has been taken-for-granted and is often overlooked. There are many studies that examine work roles, tasks and activities, the process of nursing, and problems of concern to nurses and these studies provide much useful information. However, they are not as successful in capturing the content, process and outcomes of practice as are those studies which take an interpretative approach to examine practice as it is experienced by nurses. In order to adequately understand the nature of everyday experience in practice and how it contributes to the development of expertise, it is important to capture the contextual, relational, and complex yet particular nature of everyday nursing practice. Before turning to the ward sisters' everyday nursing practice, however, it is necessary to look first at the complex nature of the ward sisters' experience itself. The next four chapters are a discussion of the nature of experience, the nature of ward sister practice, the context of that experience, and an exploration of the process of practising nursing and of becoming experienced. They are based upon the interviews and periods of participant observation, during which I shadowed the Ward Sisters in the course of their daily work.

4

Experience as movement

INTRODUCTION

In the course of my interviews with the Ward Sisters, the Sisters described in some detail their experiences in nursing and of people they had nursed. As I shadowed them in practice, they would sometimes comment on what they were doing, either spontaneously or in response to a question from either myself or a student. Perhaps what is most striking to me from their accounts is how elusive and fluid experience seems to be and how much of their everyday practice is taken for granted and is therefore missing from the accounts. From this, it appears that the notion of experience is not as straightforward as it first seems and as it is often portrayed in the literature. Experience happens in the midst of time; it is imbued with meaning. Sometimes experience is understood to be intensely personal, yet at the same time we talk about sharing an experience with others. It would appear that the temporal nature of experience, its meaningfulness and its personal yet contextual nature, all contribute to its complexity and elusiveness. This chapter concerns the problematic nature of experience and how experience manifests itself in the accounts and practices of the Sisters.

THE PROBLEM WITH EXPERIENCE

Before I examine the Sisters' accounts of their experiences it would be helpful to turn again to the experiential learning models first introduced in Chapter 2. These models were shown to treat experience as a relatively non-problematic entity, a source for learning. By examining some of their features in depth, we are better able to see some of the problems with experience itself.

Time and meaning in experience

The experiential learning models (Lewin 1952, Revans 1980, Kolb 1984, Boud et al 1985, Jarvis 1987a, Jarvis 1992) perhaps show most clearly that when experience is conceptualized as an atemporal event it can be isolated, described and reflected upon. In this analysis, experience 'consists of the total response of a person to a situation or event: what he or she thinks, feels, does and concludes at the time and immediately thereafter' (Boud et al 1985 p 18). It can be recalled that in the experiential learning models, experiences are presented as but one discrete stage of a serial, circular process (Figure 4.1). Although the specifics of the models differ considerably, their basic stages are similar to those first outlined by Lewin (1952) and adopted most directly by Kolb (1984).

The experiential learning theorists take the view that experiences do not have value in and of themselves, but are a source of concepts or material for reflection. Experiences are essentially atemporal — moments in time which can be isolated, held in the memory and recaptured when needed. They are like events which fill up spaces in time.

The problems with this approach show up most clearly in Jarvis' (1987a, 1992) model as he addresses the issue of everyday experiences. Unlike other experiential learning theorists who

merely acknowledge everyday experiences and concentrate on eventful experiences which can be described, Jarvis (1987a, 1987b, 1992) suggests that everyday experiences can be accounted for by considering their meaningfulness. Meaning, in his model, is conferred upon experiences which have passed (Jarvis 1987a pp 72–77). He uses the term, biography, to describe the memories of all a person's experiences, which are brought to bear when a person apprehends social situations, thus changing the situations into experiences. Everyday experiences which cause minimal or no disjuncture between a situation and a biography are meaningful if reflection can be prompted, and meaningless when the content of the experience does not prompt reflection. What remains problematic in this approach is that it assumes that a person can be in situations which are devoid of meaning and that meaning can be conferred upon some periods of existence and withheld from others.

Considering experiences as if they were atemporal events raises the serious question of what is happening in people's lives when situations or experiences do not count as discrete events. What happens in the taken-for-granted everyday flow of life which makes up the majority of our existence?

Researchers working within an interpretative or hermeneutic phenomenological approach face different problems related to time and meaning. Notably, problems with meaning concern the meaningful nature of experience and the understanding of meaning itself. Commonly in everyday life we talk about sharing experiences through conversation, a joke, or perhaps even a glance. That is not to say that when experiences are shared they are understood in exactly the same way by each of the participants. However, such commonality of understanding in our practices and language points to shared background meanings which already exist in our experiences and which can be revealed through interpretation (Heidegger 1962). This perspective holds that no experience is meaningless but there are some experiences which may be imbued with more meaning than others. In this vein, following Gadamer's (1975 p 317) notion of '"experience" in the real sense'

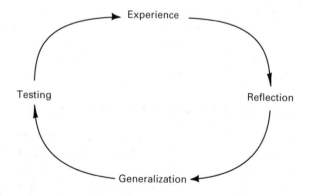

Figure 4.1 Experiential learning process

as always being a negation of prior under-standing, Benner (1984) selects for analysis those experiences which stand out in a nurse's mind as having affected her and her practice.

In hermeneutic phenomenology, the temporality of experienced situations is depicted as directional and relational (Heidegger 1962). That is, experienced situations always take place in a flow of time. Time shows up, or is manifested in relation to the context of the situation. Unlike conventional accounts which use the metaphor of space to depict time as discrete serial events, Heidegger uses the metaphor of activity to express temporality. When time is understood as activity, the rhythmic or temporal nature of experience is seen to be important (Clandinin 1989). The timing, pacing and flow of action and experience is recognized. It is exceedingly difficult to capture the actual temporal nature of the experience however, when experiences are transposed into verbal or textual narratives. Nuances of timing and pacing — crucial components in the meanings of everyday human actions — can only be pointed to in descriptions of experience: they cannot be completely captured.

Although the location of meaning and the temporal sense differ markedly between the experiential learning models and the interpretative/hermeneutic phenomenological approach, the question still arises, 'What is happening in the taken-for-granted flow of life as it relates to experience?'.

Telling about experience

In the experiential learning models, experience is essentially thought to consist of raw data: it provides the basis for reflection and the place for assimilating or using newly formed concepts. Boud (1987) suggests that reflection is the way in which learners '... process the experiences they have ...' (p 233). In considering experience to be an event made up of raw data, the models suggest that experience is straightforward; something which can be recalled as a piece by an individual. A particular experience can be replayed in the mind's eye and such replaying becomes the first stage of reflection. For instance, in an educational context, a person is asked to 'return' to the experience:

... to recall in detail exactly what happened: who they met, who said what, how each person reacted, what they felt at each point in time, what occupied their attention, what else was going on. The idea is to recapture, in as much detail as possible, the full experience of the event and the reactions of all those associated with it. (Boud 1987 p 233)

Implied here is the fact that experiences are lying as entities in a person's memory and are there to be recaptured. Yet whilst recalling experiences in some detail would indeed appear to be feasible, as can be seen from the Sisters' accounts of their experiences, it seems unlikely that the recall can be as complete as Boud suggests. The notion of 'the full experience' is rather misleading. As we go through life, we are tacitly aware of more than can be accounted for in verbal reconstructions of experiences (Polanyi [1958]1962). In telling about any experience, we can relay only a portion of what was going on at the time. It is illusory to think that the entirety of an experience could ever be re-created through retrospection, even though accounts do provide a fruitful source of understandings, meanings and practices.

This view of experience as a discrete event, a collection of data which can be retrieved as it was deposited and then processed, also belies the interpretative nature of experience. It suggests that there is a subjective reality to an experience and that the experience will be recounted in the same way each time it is recalled. This view would have us believe that the situation which provokes the recollection, as well as any intervening experience, do not influence what is recalled, nor how it is recalled. Such a view also points towards a notion of subjective experience in which experiences are only revealed by what an individual says about them.

The interpretative character of experience and recollection is also overlooked when it is suggested that one can 'refrain from making judgements' in describing experience (Boud et al 1985 p 27). It fails to recognize that even in the act of describing or telling, the language used reveals the person's interpretation of the experience and judgements about what to tell and how to tell it.

The interpretative nature of accounts of experiences are recognized more explicitly by researchers using hermeneutic phenomenological approaches who attempt to understand the meanings and 'meaning structures' of experiences as they are lived. Descriptions of a particular situation or event as it is lived are used as the source of understanding (Benner 1984, van Manen 1984). Such situations or events are usually in the past, although sometimes actual, ongoing practices are included. Descriptions of experiences are usually gathered or created in the form of narratives, schemes 'for linking individual human actions and events into interrelated aspects of an understandable composite' (Polkinghorne 1988 p 13). This approach does not claim a direct correlation between the narrative and the actual experience, rather narratives are held to provide insight into the experience as well as to give form and meaning to the experience itself (Polkinghorne 1988, Allen et al 1989). The central role played by language is acknowledged. Missing from these researchers' works, however, is an examination of the form in which experience is expressed. The narrative form is taken as usual and unproblematic. It is further assumed that the emotions felt by the person during the experience can and will be expressed.

The temporal nature of experience is revealed in the way we speak about experiencing. For ourselves, and for the Sisters in the study whose experience I will explore shortly, everyday experience is spoken about as something fluid, in the past as well as in the present. However, when we talk about our 'experience' it is usually of experiences which have already happened and which have stood out enough to be remembered. We seldom consider ourselves to be experiencing in present, 'real' time. This is perhaps because we take this for granted, and only talk about experience when we stop to actively reflect on what has already happened. Experience as we live it on a moment-to-moment basis is seldom narrated in the form in which it is actually experienced. We make leaps forwards and backwards, making connections between the past and the present and among experiences in the past. Connections which we actually make

between past experience and present action can only be guessed at, and can only be incompletely described. Indeed, the Sisters often found it impossible to make a concrete link between their current practices and experiences which had informed them. They recognized, however, that real but tacit links existed.

The largely non-verbal nature of many practices also poses a problem for the depiction of experiences. Whilst we may have many experiences we put into words, there are many others that we cannot even come close to describing fully with words. Consider the feeling of hitting a golf ball just right, the smell of bread baking, or the feeling when a close friend dies. Words which are available to us often are inadequate to describe such bodily and qualitative distinctions in experiences. This inability to completely capture nuances of everyday practices and experiences points to the difficulty of describing experience, both past and ongoing, and to understanding connections within experience.

Given these problems: of understanding the nature of everyday experience; understanding the relationship between experience as people live it and how they tell about it; and the difficulties in capturing experience as it is happening, what can one say about the experiences of nurses in everyday practice?

It seems from the literature, and from observing and listening to the Sisters that nurses concomitantly draw upon experience and add to it whilst they work. Their everyday practices form the basis of their experiences. At the same time, they are adding to their experience whilst they are practising nursing. Even though it seems impossible to completely capture experience, it seems possible to capture something of everyday nursing by examining ongoing practices as well as accounts of experiences in practice.

CAPTURING THE SISTERS' EXPERIENCE

Before going on to explore the Sisters' experiences, it is useful to describe the nature of the data on which the following discussions are based. When the research started, it was my intention that the interviews would be foreground or primary data. The material arising from the participant observations would be background material, used only as a way of understanding the context within which the Sisters practised. I felt the observations were necessary to become familiar with practices, organizational constraints and opportunities which informed the Sisters' accounts of their experiences. They would assist a meeting of 'horizons' during the interpretation.

The problems inherent in understanding experiences from narrative accounts soon became apparent. There were marked discrepancies between the accounts and the fullness of the Sisters' everyday practice. The accounts were consistent with what I observed them doing: the picture of the Sisters' practice which came across in the interviews was very similar to the picture I saw in everyday practice. However, there were many things happening in practice which I found to be remarkable yet which the Sisters found commonplace and not worth a mention.

The difficulty of describing connections between past and current experiences also became apparent as the Sisters had great difficulties telling how they came to be able to do some of the things they found to be commonplace. 'Just experience' was often the response. Seldom did the Sisters report that they drew on whole situations as they met current situations as Benner (1984) postulates. More often, connections between the past and present were contained within a look, a phrase, a feeling, or something they could not describe beyond 'experience'.

The form of the narratives

The shape and character of the Sisters' narrative accounts of past experiences are also different from those reported by Diekelmann (1989), Benner (1984) and others undertaking research using the 'significant experience' interview guide (see Appendix 1). Unlike those researchers, I was able to gather few well-formed narratives, 'paradigm cases', but the Sisters did talk at length about memorable patients and experiences. It was sometimes difficult to get the 'full' situation in a coherent, narrative form, including many

details about what was going on at the time and how the Sister was feeling. The Sisters also had great difficulty telling me about a time in which they 'made a difference' to a patient. At the same time, the difference which their care made to patients was evident (and recognized by the Sisters) in their discussions and ongoing practice.

It is difficult to extract the possible reasons for the differences in the form of narratives between this research and that of Benner and Diekelmann, but the differences point towards possible features of the Sisters' experience. One feature is the influence of culture. The form of the accounts about experience may have been influenced by what is often called 'Scottish reticence'. When asked to tell me about a situation in which she made a difference to a patient, one Sister said, 'It sounds awful boasty, this, Martha' (Int. 4-1: 1).

Unlike American nurses, whose culture and educational programmes encourage them to relate experiences in some detail, Scottish nurses are not used to doing this. Even in educational situations, nurses are often reluctant to talk about experiences that they consider to be minor, or experiences which they think the listeners would have experienced themselves. Teachers of nursing not only find students reluctant to bring experiences to share in seminars, they sometimes also find it difficult to get students to discuss experiences in sufficient detail to be able to examine the significant features (Stewart E, personal communication 1990). Other researchers have noted similar differences between Americans and Scots in reporting and addressing feelings in health care situations (Strong 1979).

A second feature is the effect of experience itself. As will be discussed shortly, the form of the narrative appears to be related to the nature of the experience. The Sisters related remarkably few 'firsts', such as a first death, or other dramatic, moving stories. I focused more on recent experiences in the second and third interviews, seeking links with everyday practice and, because of this, there were fewer emotionally charged, fully expressed experiences than perhaps there might have been had I persisted in seeking critical incidents (Flanagan 1954). In contrast, Benner concentrates on events which stand out for nurses whilst placing a much smaller emphasis on moment-by-moment, taken-for-granted experiences (Benner 1984, 1991, Benner & Wrubel 1989).

Insights into experience

The Sisters' accounts cannot be said to completely reflect their experience because feelings may not be expressed fully, and details may be a fraction of what went on. Nevertheless, some insights into experience are certainly gained. Experience is fluid and much of it remains hidden, thereby making it impossible to entirely indicate its features. However, the interviews give insights into the Sisters' experiences of practice in the past, their comments on recent practice and connections which they are able to make (or not able to make) between current and past practices.

When observing practice, I can presume that experience is being drawn upon, but I cannot see the potential in the current situation which is there to be drawn upon. Indeed, neither can the Sisters. They cannot say what of their current experience may ultimately be drawn upon, nor how it will be drawn upon. In other words, they cannot determine what aspects of today's practice will join that ever-changing, amorphous body that they refer to as their 'experience'. Although there are some exceptions, both the Sisters and I have difficulty identifying when in their current practice they are drawing on past experience. The connection is not and cannot be entirely clear. Having said that, what I do have in the field notes are insights into how the Sisters are working, their comments on their current practice, and what their current nursing practice looks like. Importantly, I have been able to capture something of the flow of practice over a few days at a time.

The interviews and observations allow the unexamined — what experience means to these Sisters and how practice and experience move together — to be examined. In looking at how they currently practice, and in hearing about their experience, I am speculating that the Sisters are drawing on something, that they are drawing on it in particular ways, and that *it* came from something not unlike the practice I saw.

WHAT COUNTS AS EXPERIENCE

Two ways of understanding experience emerge from the Sisters' descriptions. One is of experience as an entity, a possession of the person, 'the experience that you've gained . . .' (Int. 5-3: 31); 'I don't have enough staffing, that is, experienced staff' (W9D2-1: 17). This sense of 'experience' is captured, for the most part, in retrospective accounts of experiences, and occasionally in present actions or future intentions: '[Y]ou can get that experience today. It is good to get it early in your training' (W7D2-1: 8). This sense of 'experience' is a result of the process of 'experiencing' (Gadamer 1975 pp 316–317).

'Experiencing' expresses the other way of understanding experience: experience as an ongoing process, of acting in a situation, in an historical time and place; it could be said to be the process of being. This sense of experience, I suggest, is best expressed as *experience as movement*, as it encompasses both ongoing, dynamic activity as well as a change in the person. In this vein, Sr Aitkin talks of '. . . the experience of talking to people' (Int. 1-3: 47).

Experience in the first sense, experience which we possess because we have had it, grows out of the second, experience as a process. However, it is not as simple as saying one is in the present and the other is in the past, nor saying one is a product and the other is a process. The two are intertwined. It seems that experience which we have had is not static, but is in continual flux; it is inseparable from experiencing the present. This emerges in the Sisters' discussions of their experiences, as well as in their everyday practice.

The process of experience is revealed through examining moment-by-moment practice and the connections between experience and experiencing. As a process, experience involves learning. In Gadamer's explanation of experience as the turning around of preconception, learning is presumed in the motion whereby previous experience is negated by new experience (Gadamer 1975). He does not address learning directly. Benner (1984) and Dreyfus & Dreyfus (1986) also address learning obliquely[1]. The Sisters, however, talk directly about learning in practice. In their experiences, learning appears to be conterminous with experiencing as well as being an outgrowth of experience.

What counts as experience then is experience as movement: the process of experiencing in addition to experience as a result or event. Both senses of experience emerge in the interviews and observations. Before moving on to the features of experiences and experiencing, it may be useful to explore how experiences are revealed in the Sisters' accounts and practice.

Unlike the unitary picture of experience which emerges in Benner's exemplars or paradigm cases (Benner 1984, 1987), and in the writing of the experiential learning theorists, the Sisters' experiences take many forms. They are not all 'of a piece' within a defined time frame. Some are all of a piece, but more often they are more amorphous and discontinuous. Their experience can not be neatly categorized. However, the following examples and descriptions are presented to show something of the diversity.

'I've never forgotten': watershed experience

Watershed experiences are unforgettable experiences which stand out in the Sisters' minds. They are Benner's paradigm cases. In the following interview excerpt, Sr Jarvis describes an experience in which she learns about the early warning signs of a serious postoperative complication.

Sr Jarvis: I remember quite clearly a patient who went into clot retention after a prostatectomy. And this is quite a long time ago because it was when I was a staff nurse in the unit, when I was quite junior at the time. And this was something that worried me greatly because there was no one else around to whom I could turn. No other staff nurse and no sister.

And this man's catheter wasn't draining and I had to try to wash it out and couldn't get anywhere with it at all. Couldn't get anything in or out and the patient was in EXTREME pain. I very soon realized that I wasn't going to be able to do anything that would make any difference at all. So we phoned to theatre to ask to speak to a doctor because the Resident wasn't around. And the Registrar came to see him. And he tried to wash the catheter out as well and decided that there was no way we were getting anywhere and he'd have to go back to theatre.

But it was something that I've never forgotten because it brought home to me very clearly how important it was that these catheters drained after theatre and how very quickly if they didn't, you'd end up with a patient that had a bladder full of clot that was going to have to go back to theatre and have another operation to remove it. And it's something that ever since, I feel I'm always emphasizing to the nurses how they MUST watch the catheters' draining, how they MUST make sure the irrigation is always running and never never stopped. And because of that, having seen what can happen if it doesn't.

M.M.: Mmm. Can you tell me what happened up until that point that affected you so much?

Sr Jarvis: I think because for the first time ... I was expected to know what to do. It had been the first situation where I didn't know how to cope. And I couldn't just turn to somebody and say, 'I'm not happy about this; what do you think?' I had to decide that this was far from right and that somebody, medical staff would have to come and see it.

M.M.: ... Do you remember what other staff was on that night?

Sr Jarvis: I don't remember exactly who was on with me but they were obviously students for there to be no other qualified nurse about. And obviously they wouldn't be expected to know any better than me about that sort of thing. It was specialized.

I think you always feel protected and then all of a sudden there has to be a situation where YOU have to make the decision. It's lucky you know enough how to do it when it comes.[laugh] But you don't get trained for it.

M.M.: No. Do you remember how you felt at the time?

Sr Jarvis: Extremely anxious. And when I had spoken to the doctor on the phone I then went back to the patient to make sure that it WAS necessary for him to come and I wasn't making a fuss. Because I was quite new and I didn't want to look to be stupid.

So of course I was then extremely relieved [laugh]. To find out that there wasn't something that I could have done anything about.

M.M.: Right ... Have you been in situations since ... where that has been brought back to you?

Sr Jarvis: I've been in several situations since whereby I knew that if we didn't watch very carefully this same thing would happen to this patient as it happened to another one.

And I've also come close. I think two patients since have, in fact, been in clot retention and ... I've had the medical attention far quicker than when I first had to deal with it. (Int. 10-1: 6–9)

This experience speaks of several things for Sr Jarvis. First, it is an experience of coming to know about a specific aspect of nursing care in her specialty. She is also learning about herself in practice. For Sr Jarvis this experience speaks of gaining confidence in her perceptual abilities and in her capability to make important clinical decisions on her own. She learns that her judgement is sound; she does not call the doctor unnecessarily. Second, she learned specific skills from this experience early in her practice which she continues to use as she copes with similar patients, monitoring them closely and intervening more rapidly. Although she would have known about postoperative bleeding before, Sr Jarvis can pinpoint this situation as the beginning of her current know-how regarding taking action. Third, it is a first experience, one in which Sr Jarvis has responsibility and has to make a decision. At the time, she is in her first ward as a qualified nurse. The experience is emotionally charged; Sr Jarvis' anxiety comes through. Fourth, this experience stands out. She has vivid, specific memories of a particular situation. Her account of the experience is specific, full and lucid. What Sr Jarvis has learned from this experience has stayed with her. It is noticeable in her current practice, particularly in how she guides students in monitoring patients.

Watershed experiences are related by all of the Sisters in the interviews, usually during the first and second interviews. As the Sister relates them, the context is full and the telling is lucid. These experiences have most likely been told before. One Sister describes them as 'stories'. The time frame is exact. The Sister places the experience in relation to where she was at the time. Many such situations occur in the early part of a Sister's career: during training, in the first staff nurse job, the first time in a new clinical area or early in the experience of being a ward sister. The experience usually occurs over a relatively short period of time, within a shift or at most, over a few days. The topic of the experience is significant. Often, it is the first time the Sister encounters something, for example, her first death. Sometimes, it is of a magnitude she has never experienced before, or has not expected to encounter, for example a horrendous gangrenous wound developing from a rectal abscess (Int. 9-2: 1–3). Usually, it is a situation in which the Sister's understanding is radically challenged.

Typically, the experience is emotionally charged. This comes across in the telling, even though the situation may have happened decades before, such as seeing a child die for the first time (Int. 4-1: 20). Often the feeling is one of high anxiety, and is linked to feelings of not coping. Occasionally, there is a feeling of joy and great pleasure, when, for the first time, something that has been a struggle before comes smoothly and really goes well. In the accounts, the Sister focuses on herself, how she feels, and what impact the situation is having on her. That is not to say that she does not describe the situation vividly. Often small details are included, like the colour of a person's eyes or hair.

For the most part, the meaning for the Sister of watershed situations lies in a change in her understanding: she is brought face to face with her own competence or incompetence; she realizes the importance of an aspect of care she took for granted or was unaware of before; she understands the impact her actions can have on a patient; she realizes the effect a patient can have on herself. Many of these experiences concern discrete skills or are the beginning or early part of gaining a complex skill. Sometimes the experiences stand on their own, but often the Sisters consciously make links between these experiences and their current practice.

'It comes running back to me': resonant experience

When asked to relate specific experiences, the majority of experiences related by the Sisters were resonant experiences. Some of these were told during the first interview, the majority of the second and third interviews consisted of resonant experiences. In many instances they take the form of experiences with memorable patients, or with patients currently or recently in the ward. Other times, they take the form of experiences with staff members, doctors and others. These experiences may have taken place some years previously, but they are usually recent, within the last year or two. In many instances, the experience comes out piece-meal, often hesitantly to begin with. The Sister describes a person or a situation, but it is clear in the telling that the aspect being related is only that, one aspect of the Sister's whole experience. In these experiences, the time span varies greatly. The experience may take place within a day, over several days, or even over months. It often spans the time during which the Sister was acquainted with the patient.

The emotional content of these experiences is markedly less than that of the watershed experiences, but it is not absent. In some experiences, the Sister's discomfort or anxiety is relieved when she comes to understand the situation differently. In other experiences, the Sister's care and commitment is evident; it is sometimes accompanied by sadness, pleasure or satisfaction.

In these resonant experiences, the Sister is coping smoothly; she is confident in her practice but is often wrestling with a nursing problem. Her focus is outside herself, on the patient or her colleagues. Details of the experience concern the relationships between people or aspects of the particular problem. Often the meaning of the situation for the Sister lies in how patients and their families cope with illness. It also may be an insight gained gradually over time about her own practice. The Sisters sometimes say, 'I finally realized'. Sometimes embedded in the situation are understandings which the Sisters may not have thought about before, perhaps because they have not felt the need, or because the opportunity has not been there to relate the experience as a whole.

In the following interview excerpt, Sr Baxter makes a connection between a 'resonant experience' and a taken-for-granted practice. The taken-for-granted practice falls within the next group of experiences, the 'bits and bobs', which form the majority of everyday experience. In this excerpt, it is easy to see how difficult it is to grasp ongoing experience and to make definitive links within experience. Sr Baxter describes her experience of timing and pacing a conversation with a 'difficult' patient, Mrs Harriet Harrison[2]. The conversation took place the previous day and was only discussed because I questioned her about it. For ease of reading, the excerpt has been edited.

M.M.: [. . .] You just took your time to do it. Were you aware of that at the time?
Sr Baxter: Un hun. Probably. I would get some

responses from the way Harriet looks.
Oh you can tell. She smiles sometimes. Sometimes she looks a bit, not strange, a bit more um positive when she's determined not to do something. Or you can tell the look of determination. That means she's got what she wants to do on her mind. And when [. . .] I see it coming or I see that look of questioning on her face then I know that that's enough. I know that I don't go any further.
It's like this morning when she wouldn't take her medicines. [. . .] She was taking tiny wee sips. And if I had forced it she wouldn't have touched it at all. I think now, that's the feeling I got.
That if I pushed through then she would just say, 'Well I'm not . . .' She would begin to use her adjectives again. 'I'm not going to take it.' And [. . .] I think she wouldn't have touched it. So it's better to let her do it in her own time. (Int. 2-3: 5–6)

In this experience, Sr Baxter attends carefully to Mrs Harrison's face and notices her responses. Sr Baxter gets feedback on her actions, understands the meaning of Mrs Harrison's responses and alters her actions to meet them. She has not always had this ability. She remembers not having it when she was a qualified staff nurse of about 5 years experience, newly working in the neurosurgical unit.

Sr Baxter: [. . .] And I hadn't long been there and insisting that patients must take their medicine. You sign for them [. . .] to say that they've taken them and if the patient hasn't taken them, you've signed it. So that in effect is wrong.
[. . .] And there used to be patients who [. . .] became quite restless because of their illness and you couldn't reason with them. Somehow these patients had to get their medicines. And I felt that I had this right for the patient to take it whether they wanted it or not.
M.M.: Mm hmm. Can you remember . . . that turning point for you?
Sr Baxter: . . . . I can't. I can't say that it is something that's quite foremost in my mind. [. . .]
But that turning point came in dealing with people who were agitated: whom you couldn't communicate with as easily as, I suppose, as with Harriet. [. . .] Somehow over that period I came to the, not conclusion, but I understood that people were people. And that you had to go with them as people. And that you've got 20 people on the ward and they're all different. And whilst you can't have routines for every one of them to suit their own individual needs you've got to try, and to a certain extent go with them.
[. . .] I'm aware of it happening. I don't know when. But I'm aware of now being different from how I used to be in that respect. And I think that was when I realized that they were people. And it didn't matter

because you've signed a piece of paper, as long as they took it. [. . .]

And there were some situations you approached . . . differently from others. And I — I don't know. That's something that I . . . sensed. You know sometimes that if there is somebody who won't do anything, you've got to be firm. And maybe had Gladys [another 'particular' patient on the ward] been here for longer and she wasn't going to take her medicine, then that for the long term couldn't persist. And you'd have to think of some plan to help her.

And it may be that you would have to be a wee bit more . . . . um . . . forthright in some things, in some respects. And give them leeway in others. Because over a long period of time maybe that wouldn't be the approach every time. (Int. 2-3: 6–8)

Sr Baxter's experience of coming to know people as people could be interpreted as an odd experience to have 5 years after qualification. The nursing textbooks stress that nurses should treat the person as an individual and the Sisters endorse this general principle.

However, this 'resonant experience' reveals something of the deepening of understanding, not only of coming to know people as individuals, but also of practising from that understanding, particularly in complex circumstances. This example speaks of coming to a new way of knowing-in-practice. Sr Baxter does not throw away the textbook knowledge of medication administration, but looks beneath and beyond to something more complex — to what is possible in order to care for the person in a way which most suits that person. Her focus moves from concern about her practice to looking through her practice directly to the patient. Sr Baxter is telling about changing to a flexible stance. It started with the issue of giving medications to brain-injured patients, and has gradually become part of her practice with all patients. Up until this point for Sr Baxter, caring about the person was one aspect (amongst many) of what she was trying to achieve. Her change of focus depicts a qualitative leap in her practice. She becomes able to approach the person as an individual; it now suffuses everything she does. It is evident in her style of practice, which is often one of negotiation. Her practice presumes a trust and respect of the person.

Her description is quite different from Sr Jarvis' description of her experience. Firstly, unlike Sr Jarvis who centres on a specific aspect of her practice, Sr Baxter's experience concerns a more far-reaching change. Sr Baxter recognizes a change in herself. '[I am] different from how I used to be.' Changes in a specific area of practice may indeed prompt changes in other areas because of an increase in confidence, for example. On the other hand, a change in oneself, such as Sr Baxter describes, differently enframes all of her future practice.

Secondly, whilst Sr Jarvis recognizes the experience as a time of specific change, Sr Baxter doesn't remember changing: she only remembers when she was not as flexible. She relates it to a time when she was having difficulty with an inflexible response, but not to a particular patient situation. I can presume that in the neurosurgery ward more than one patient did not cooperate with nursing care.

Thirdly, Sr Baxter does not relate the experience as a first time event. She was already a seasoned staff nurse. Fourthly, the situation and process are not easily told and are not 'something that's quite foremost in my mind'. In telling me about it, Sr Baxter hesitates and repeats herself. Her sentences are not as fluid as they often are. Her experiences of people have prompted a subtle but important change in her understanding of people, in her understanding of interactions with them, and in her understanding of herself. It has taken place over time and is not easy to describe. It has come:

With experience. Just with dealing with people like Harriet and Gladys that are quite determined in their own way. In the end I found out that you know, you don't go in . . . You, you get more by going at their pace. (Sr Baxter Int. 2-3: 6)

'Just the bits and bobs': taken-for-granted experience

'Bits and bobs', taken-for-granted experiences which happen all the time in everyday practice make up, by far, the majority of nursing experience. However, the Sisters talk about these experiences only in the field notes and during the third interviews with each Sister when I asked them about specific aspects of their practice which I had observed. They are the recent and 'real-time' experiences. Often what I had observed in detail is related by them in the broadest of terms: 'just a routine day', 'just an exploratory conversation'. Rarely is there a more detailed description of the complex interactions I observed. Sometimes, the Sisters had forgotten the occasion, but more frequently, it had not stood out enough to talk about it, except in the context of a question on another subject.

The time frames of the experiences are momentary, a scrap of conversation, a comment, even a look. However, they are embedded in broader experiences of relationships with patients and colleagues. The emotional levels of these experiences vary, with calmness, 'the usual' frustration, sadness, puzzlement and pleasure all being among the emotions expressed. The Sisters are all coping in these experiences with a greater or lesser degree of comfort. When the Sisters tell about these experiences, the focus is rarely on themselves, on their own experience and feelings. They play only an incidental part. The focus is on the patient or colleagues and their responses in particular situations. The meaning of the experience primarily lies in practice, in understanding patients and how to accomplish the work of the ward.

Through these 'bits and bobs', taken-for-granted experiences, the Sisters' skills and understandings are reinforced, extended and refined. They form and transform the Sisters' everyday practice, but are usually hidden, appearing only in discussion at handover report or during informal discussions among nurses. Some may come to light, however, when the understanding arising from these everyday practices and taken-for-granted knowledge comes to a point that it forms a new whole, and the Sister expresses it as an experience which resonates with her.

Thus far in the discussion, different kinds of experiences have been distinguished. I have suggested that experiences take many forms and have delineated three kinds of experiences to demonstrate the range.

1. *Watershed* experiences, which are vivid, highly memorable, emotionally charged, and specifically meaningful for the Sisters, and often concern first-time situations.
2. *Resonant* experiences, which are less emotionally charged, are the result of cumulated, taken-for-granted experience, often focus on patients or a gradual change in self-understanding and need prompting to be recalled.
3. *'Bits and bobs'*, the taken-for-granted experiences which happen all the time, have a relatively even emotional tone, concern the ongoing practising of the Sisters, are often forgotten soon afterwards or are not considered to be important enough to tell about.

I have further proposed that experience has to do with change, with the deepening and broadening of the Sister's understanding of herself, her patients and her practice. In the next sections, aspects of the ground of experience as movement will be excavated[3].

AWARENESS OF EXPERIENCE

A question which remains unaddressed in both the experiential learning literature and the phenomenological literature on nursing experience concerns people's awareness of their everyday experiences in practice. How aware are the Sisters of their ongoing experience?

In many instances, the Sisters are conscious of their experiences and the changes in understanding which accompany them. This is particularly so with 'watershed' experiences which prompt sudden insight. Through the experience reported on p 45, Sr Jarvis becomes aware of her new understanding of a particular postoperative complication, the development of a clot in the bladder, and how it presents in the patient. Although she does not explicitly state it, Sr Jarvis newly recognizes her powers of assessment. Her confidence increases and in subsequent situations, 'I knew... that this same thing would happen...' Her experience in the earlier situation prompts her to notice and act differently. In a subsequent situation (Int. 10-1:

9–10) she realizes with the 'first syringe of water' that she is facing a forming clot, and so gets the Registrar 'to come and see him'. Her prompt action averts the need for the patient to return to theatre. Experiences in subsequent, similar situations confirm her understanding and actions, and reinforce her confidence in her perceptions.

At other times, the Sisters are not explicitly aware of their experiences. Such experiences confirm previous experience, or encompass subtle or imperceptible changes; prompting awareness only when the accumulated movement is significant, or a new situation calls forth a response from the Sister that she did not realize she had. Awareness of an earlier change may only come in retrospect; however, that does not mean that they have not experienced at the time. The 'bits and bobs' experiences, in particular, throw into question Benner's (1984) contention that experience is the active '... refinement of preconceived notions and theory...' rather than the '... mere passage of time...' (p 36)[4]. The Sisters are engaged in many aspects of practice upon which they may not actively reflect but which form part of their experience. The way in which this occurs is discussed throughout Chapters 5, 6 and 7.

Frequently, the Sisters are not aware of their practices until they are called upon to tell about them. Such telling can prompt a sudden insight. Sr Fraser slows her pace to watch a patient walk down the hallway, moving slowly and holding onto the wall (W6D4: 8). My asking a question about what she is thinking prompts reflection on her practice.

Sr Fraser: I didn't even know I was doing it. [. . .] I'd never realized that you're automatically assessing them all the time. You're not even thinking about it. You're doing it. (Int. 6-3: 33–34)

Since my questioning her, Sr Fraser is 'now doing it consciously'. She contends that knowing her practice has '... not made any difference to the outcome...' or changed her practice. However, being aware of her practice allows her to point out to students the effectiveness of judging a patient's progress. She tells them, '... just watch them on their own when they're not [aware]' (Int. 6-3: 35). While she watches the patient in the hallway, Sr Fraser notices and understands the meaning of the patient's gait and comportment in terms of her progress towards recovery from ear surgery. She is experiencing the woman and the situation. Reflecting on her practice affords Sr Fraser a *new* experience, of coming to be more aware of her own practice.

The Sisters are experiencing all the time, even in conversations which quickly fade from memory and may not be called forth later in reflection. Sr Baxter's conversation with Harriet is a good example (p 47). She notices Harriet throughout the conversation and her understanding of Harriet deepens. Her experience of the conversation also confirms her knowledge about an effective approach to take with Harriet. In such low key situations, which form the majority of experiences, the Sisters' understanding is confirmed, extended and refined. While they may not be particularly memorable, these taken-for-granted experiences form the basis of the 'realization' which comes 'with experience'.

Although a Sister's practice and knowledge can be made visible and differently accessible to her, this is not a prerequisite. Tacit knowledge may be refined and deepened without becoming explicit. Sr Baxter has refined her tacit knowing of Harriet's 'look of determination' to the extent that she can see it coming. It is only when she recalls the conversation in the interview that she makes the knowing explicit. Even then she calls on my shared understanding of a 'look of determination' as her tacit knowing cannot be made fully explicit. Sr Baxter's understanding of Harriet's looks will continue to be refined in further encounters with her.

Specific changes in understanding which occur during the course of a day may be quite small. They may escape notice until they accumulate enough to prompt awareness. Then the changes in understanding come to consciousness and can be named. It seems that the Sisters become aware of changes when they form a pattern, when practices are pointed out to them, or when they are reflecting on past or future action. Understanding may take a considerable time to change; the change may be tacit. Sr Baxter cannot remember when she changed her approach to people but knows that a change occurred. At a certain point she 'sensed' a need to approach situations flexibly and 'in the end' discovered 'you get more by going at their pace'.

Whether or not the Sisters are aware of specific experiences, they show a certain openness to new experience and to finding new meanings in past experiences. How this openness manifests itself will be explored in the next chapters, but it may be useful here to explore the possible ground of this openness to experience.

BEING OPEN TO EXPERIENCE

Underlying the Sisters' receptivity to experience appear to be two phenomena: one is being in a state-of-mind, or mood and the second is being attuned to the meanings in experience. They are closely linked. As Heidegger (1962) says, we are always in a mood; we are always in a state-of-mind which allows our encounters in the world to matter to us.

The role of mood and emotion

In their accounts of their experiences and in their everyday practice, the Sisters show moods: of interest, of anxiety, of surprise, of pleasure, of sadness, of frustration, of anger. We usually refer to feeling or emotion when we speak of the type and intensity of feeling of the Sisters' state-of-mind or mood. Whilst the mood may be neutral, there is never absence of emotion.

Different situations evoke emotions of varying intensity. In the accounts of first-time encounters or other 'watershed' experiences, such as Sr Jarvis', the emotional level is high. Sr Jarvis remembers being 'extremely anxious' about the patient and making a good decision and then 'extremely relieved' that she had made the right decision. As she relates the experience the intensity of her feelings at the time comes across. Her feelings vividly remain part of her experience. Such experiences are powerful and emotionally charged, often with a sense of drama. They stay in the Sisters' minds and can be recalled in great detail decades later.

Sr Dunn: But I think that these patients and other patients when you're a young student nurse must have made a great impression on you.
[. . .] Because you can still remember these instances. And I think it's just all a matter of caring really. Because you cared. It's not that you were upset. I mean you couldn't cope and you felt so sorry for them, because that's not professional. But then you're just learning to be a professional when you're a student aren't you?
[. . .] And I think it was just the fact that you cared and 'wasn't it sad really', and it just stuck in your mind. (Int. 4-2: 44)

These first experiences of coping under pressure (or not coping as the case may be) and of being very close to patients are highly memorable. Fewer such instances stand out later in the Sisters' careers.

Sr Calder: You know what I mean? The first time when these ones happened to me it meant something, because I was frightened you know, it did start the adrenalin going but ooh ....
[. . .] I don't remember it [now] in the same way at all. And you know I'm trying. (Int. 3-2: 7)

As the Sisters have more experiences and learn to cope better, fewer situations are infused with the same level of emotion. Indeed, situations which at one time were sources of great anxiety and stress are now taken for granted. The Sisters know they can cope; they have confidence in themselves. As the Sisters gain experience they may find situations frustrating or difficult but they are not as emotionally charged. That is not to say that the Sisters become less emotionally involved in their work nor that situations and patients matter less. Rather, through experience the Sisters have developed a capacity to respond differently.

In accounts of more mundane experiences, the Sisters' feelings also come through. Describing a situation in which a staff member does not arrive at work one morning, Sr Grant expresses her feelings:

Sr Grant: . . . A battle was changed by the absence of one of our staff. [. . .] It usually means that everybody will have to do a little bit more. And since we run so close to the bare minimum anyway that can be enough to make you understaffed and that's a pressure that's felt by every member of the staff. [. . .]
.... Well, it presents a feeling of frustration. Because you can't meet your ideals or even approach your ideals. (Int. 7-1: 11)

The experience is not emotionally charged, but feeling is not absent. Sr Grant is coping in the situation. By far the majority of the Sisters' experiences consist of situations such as these. Along with frustration and anxiety, pleasure and satisfaction come through in many everyday experiences. For example, warmth and comfort comes through in Sr Baxter's conversation with Harriet.

The Sisters' feelings in a particular situation arise in great part from their concern for the ward and care for the patients. While sometimes their feelings inhibit what they notice and how they act, feelings emerging from their involvement with patients and with the ward also enable the Sisters to uncover the meanings inherent in their practice experiences (see also Benner & Wrubel 1989, Benner et al 1992).

Revealing meaning in experience

Underlying the Sisters' openness to experience is the possibility of grasping meanings inherent in the situations in which they find themselves. Meaning is always there in experience — the situation always matters to us in some way and through interpretation we understand a situation *as* something (Heidegger 1962). The Sisters' descriptions and practices give the *as* an expression (Ricoeur 1978 p 154). The way in which a situation matters is revealed in the Sisters' experience through their interpretations of particular situations.

Sr Baxter's interpretation of the meanings of the situation is revealed in her account. Her interpretation is also revealed in her ongoing practice. Sr Baxter's actions flow from her interpretation of the meaning of Harriet's facial expressions. She adjusts the timing and pacing of the conversation to accommodate the meaning she is finding there. '. . . [Y]ou can tell the look of determination . . . when I see it coming . . . then I know that's enough.' Harriet's expressions and movements are salient, pointing to how she feels and what she wishes to do. Sr Baxter captures the meaning in them, understanding when Harriet begins to feel pushed and knowing what action to take.

The meanings in situations are neither absolute nor static. Over time the Sisters understand similar situations differently. Things stand out differently and the Sisters, in turn, respond differently. What is salient and meaningful changes with new experience. When Sr Jarvis knew she could recognize the early warning signals of a developing blood clot, the meaning of similar situations changed. They were not as frightening; she knew what to look for and could act to prevent them. Her first time situation still stands out with all its vividness, although the meaning she finds in it may have changed.

Sometimes, a specific experience reveals new meaning in a particular situation. When I question Sr Fraser about her thoughts while watching the patient walk, she sees new meaning in this everyday situation, not in what she is observing, but in understanding her own practice — that she does look all the time.

The reflexive nature of meaning in experience is further illustrated by Sr Calder as she tells about seeing her first bedsore, which happened within her first 2 days of practice as a junior student.

Sr Calder: There may have been some reason why he had these bedsores, but it was right down to the, Och I'm sure it was to the head of femur. It was just the most awful sore in his side. After more experience I realized that there are some of them you can't prevent. Some of the sick patients that have laid at home, come in with bedsores. And, well, it has made me more conscious of bedsores and the treatment of bedsores. (Int. 3-1: 1–2)

Part of the initial meaning to her of this experience was how neglectful the nurses could have been. She understands this differently 'after more experience' of patients coming into hospital with bedsores. There are also hints here that she acknowledges her own limitations in preventing bedsores. Sr Calder's current practice reflects a continuing concern about preventing pressure sores: she sets up formal turning schedules for patients and is particularly vigilant for signs of skin breakdown, even with patients who are on the ward for only a day or two (W3D2-1: 7).

Situations contain a complex of meanings which can be grasped by the Sister. In relating experiences of caring for elderly patients who are receiving aggressive medical treatment at cardiac arrest, Sr Calder recognizes the complexity of meanings inherent in the situation, for the doctors, the nurses and the family.

Sr Calder: I mean OK. We have got to help them to live, but we've also got to help people to die. It's part of our duty too. You know OK we save them for a week. But it's the quality of life during that week.

And what the family are going through. What are you going through yourself — nursing that old lady like that? What are you feeling about it? (Int. 3-3: 45–46)

Sr Calder's understanding of the complexities of meanings in situations like these comes from her experiences both as a nurse and as the daughter of elderly parents who have been gravely ill.

The meanings the Sisters find in practice thus come from their experience outwith nursing as well as their experience within the profession. Their openness to experience is possible because they can interpret meaning in everyday situations.

It can be seen then that the Sisters' openness to experience is grounded in their being engaged in the situation, and in their being attuned to the meanings in experiences. Engaged in the situation, the Sisters are never devoid of feelings. Their feelings for the patients, the ward and their practice help them to be attuned to the meanings in their experiences in all parts of their life. Their involvement helps them to be open to interpreting situations in new ways; it allows for discovering new possibilities and meanings. The ward situation and the patients matter to them. Indeed, as will be seen in the next two chapters, the Sisters' involvement with the patients and in ward situations makes it possible for them to practise as they do, helping the patients towards recovery and making the ward work for the patients, their families, the nurses and others.

'IT'S HAPPENING TO US ALL THE TIME': TEMPORALITY AND THE SITUATION IN EXPERIENCE

An argument has been made in favour of experience as a phenomenon with an inherent temporality. Rather than a series of discrete events in serial order, it is proposed that the interplay of time and the situation is both constitutive and evocative of experience.

Experience in time

The Sisters are experiencing minute by minute and situation by situation. This comes through in their practice and in the interviews. In telling about their experiences, the Sisters illuminate an important feature of experience: that experiences occur within different time spans. In some instances, the time span of the experience is extensive. Sr Baxter relates her experience with a patient, 'an extremely difficult person to nurse', which takes place over the course of a year (Int. 2-1: 1–10). At other times, the experience takes place over one or two days, such as Sr Calder's experience of obtaining a suitable referral to a rehabilitation facility for an elderly patient with complex physical and family needs (Int. 3-3: 7–11). An experience can also be as small as a brief conversation, a glance or a comment in passing. Sr Calder remembers her experience of hearing a staff nurse call an elderly man 'a cabbage' and the look on the man's face as 'obviously he understood exactly what was being said' (Int. 3-1: 4). Experience is both formed by the situation and contributes to the experiencing of a new situation. It is reflexive and this is highlighted by the different time-spans of experience.

Experience is neither static nor immutable. As we will see in Chapter 5, the Sisters' practice is situated in the present, comes from the understanding afforded by the past and is operating towards the future. The stream of time influences the Sisters' understanding of current experiences, how previous experiences inform that understanding and the possibilities that can be seen. In the movement of experience, different aspects of encounters with patients and others during the workday may take on new significance or may be forgotten. What is understood to be experience with a patient or in a situation, changes. It is this fluid nature of experience which makes it so hard to grasp.

Sr Calder: [. . .] . . . . I suppose it has just come over the years with experience, really. I can't . . . . I can't specifically say. (Int. 3-3: 25)

The Sisters cannot recall when they acquired much of their know-how, particularly their understanding which has been extended and deepened.

As complex understanding contains so much taken-for-granted knowledge emerging from so many experiences, the Sisters often cannot identify a single incident which changed their practice. They find it easier to identify a time when they did not have that knowledge, or when they gained an appreciation of the importance of knowing, such as when Sr Grant comes to realize the importance of her knowledge and role in medical rounds:

Sr Grant: I have a much more important role on the ward round now than I used to have. They look to me. For instance, we get to the next patient and they look to me, 'So what's new here?'.
M.M.:   Yes. Do you remember how that came to be?
Sr Grant: I don't think it happened suddenly. I think it's something that happened progressively. And I think it's a mark of mutual trust that, you know, I'm reliable and my judgement's sufficiently sound. (Int. 7-3: 22)

The Sisters can identify a point in time when they realize that they have a new understanding of a situation, such as when Sr Inglis realizes she is 'home and dry', as she begins to feel comfortable in the role of ward sister almost a year after a difficult beginning (Int. 9-3: 10–13). In their accounts and in their ongoing practice, the Sisters' experience is interlinked with particular situations.

'Patients give us experience': the role of the situation

The Sisters are in a position of having to cope with the routine and extraordinary demands throughout their shift, day after day. However, as demonstrated in Chapter 5, their focus of practice on the ward is the patient. Patients 'give' the Sisters experience (Int. 6-2: 43); they establish the context for the Sisters to experience in a situation that matters.

Most of the experiences related by the Sisters in the interviews concern patients. Many of the experiences are of memorable patients, patients with whom the Sister had a particular relationship, or from whom the Sister gained some new insight into illness or into human nature. This opportunity to be so close to patients, to be with them in times of illness, of great vulnerability and of great strength, provides much satisfaction for the Sisters. They consider it a privilege to be allowed into these spaces of people's lives.

In the interviews, the Sisters' sense of being in a place with their patients and work colleagues comes through. It is perhaps this sense of 'placeness' which best characterizes the situation of experience. It is particular and contextual. The Sisters are 'there' in the ward, with the patients and with others. When Sr Inglis says, '. . . it's happening to us ALL the time' (Int. 9-2: 14), she illuminates this characteristic of the Sisters' experience. Their experience of patients is continuous. It comes from their physical proximity with patients over time and their presence as nurses.

In their everyday work, the Sisters' own knowledge and actions are transparent to themselves. They do not see their own practice: they see the patient and the ward.

Sr Calder: I mean I think one can TELL the type of patient if you have been looking after them for years and years and more years. I think one can tell the type of patient [who] is going to be motivated to get on and get better. You know not just in this ward. In any ward. [. . .]
[In] the surgical wards — [the patient] coming in with an appendix. You knew the ones that were going to straighten up and walk or the ones that went . . . like a half-shut knife. Ones who walk to get better; ones who . . . will put an effort into it, will suffer the initial pain which there's bound to be. Until they get going again. Others of them sort of sitting down to it and holding all their muscles tightly. All. They get all sore then. And I think you can tell that type of patient in time.
[. . .] But, I suppose it's just over the years, [you] see them come and go. It's part of their character, I think that I'm seeing. It's not something I've developed. I think it's their character that I'm assessing more than anything else. (Int. 3-1: 9)

Sr Calder does not consider knowing the patients to be something that comes from herself. They show her. Through taken-for-granted experience, the Sister deepens her understanding; her focus is on the patients and their responses to illness, surgery and hospitalization.

Being in the situation makes the knowledge vivid and understood. The Sisters can know about something, but not really understand the meaning until they experience it. Sr Jarvis knows about the possibility of bladder clots, but until she is in the situation where she sees the clot forming and where she has the responsibility for acting, her understanding of the signs of clot development and of her own ability in recognizing them is incomplete. Experience means actually being in a situation, acting in a situation, feeling the emotions, noticing what happens and when it happens, and being influenced by the effect of your actions on the patient or ward.

'I had to do something about it': the interplay of responsibility and experience

Experiences which have made a great impact on the Sisters often include the issue of responsibility. When the Sister practises, she is involved with the patients and the work of the ward. They matter to her. Having responsibility and feeling the commitment of responsibility creates possibilities for action. In Sr Jarvis' example, there was '... no one else around to whom I could turn'. She had to make a decision; she had to act. For her it was the first time, 'I was expected to know what to do'. Before, she had felt protected; there were others who would take the responsibility. Although she knew '... enough how to do it ...', Sr Jarvis had not previously had to make this kind of crucial decision by herself. Taking action because she *had* to transformed her understanding and her confidence.

Not only in first time experiences is responsibility pivotal. Responsibility inherent in her position prompts the Ward Sister to produce alternative approaches to problems which arise in the ward.

Sr Baxter: [...] [W]hen you then become the manager and the senior one and you have to do something about it. If you're aiming to do something about it, it's not as easy as you sometimes think.

And then you think, 'Well, what am I going to do about it?' And I suppose from that point, you start and sometimes you look at things differently, you know. And maybe as a junior or a staff nurse, you always knew there was somebody else there, that you could hand it over to. And when that responsibility is yours, you see things differently. I mean, you can't just walk away and leave them.

That's not to say that you can always fix every problem that comes your way. I mean sometimes

there are no answers. And you've got to do your best and you've got to learn to live with that. You learn to cope with it. And you learn to cope with it because you are in the situation. (Int. 2-3: 26–27)

Having responsibility prompts the Sister to act, and to consider the situation and its possibilities and limitations. Even extensive clinical practice opportunities in basic or post-basic education courses may not be as meaningful as the experience which follows. Sr Fraser tells about how her experience now is more meaningful because she has responsibility and is in situations in which '... basically all the care goes down to you' (Int. 6-1: 15). Having responsibility engages the Sisters. It commits them to action and by acting in concrete situations, they experience.

THE ROLE OF CONFIDENCE IN EXPERIENCE

Characteristically, the Sisters all have confidence in their perceptions and in their practice. Theirs is not bravado but a quiet confidence born of experience and transformative of present experience. Confidence both comes from experience and forms experience, and this movement of experience is most evident in the Sisters' discussions of confidence. Part of practising with confidence is drawing on past experience.

Drawing on experience: experience as a resource

Implied in the movement of experience, is movement from one place to another. Experience as a resource speaks of the place from which experience moves and is revealed in the Sisters' discussions of situations in which they knew what to do. Experience is part of you, forming the horizon of your understanding. Sr Ellis' comment, '... you're looking out of practice' reflects this notion. As a resource, experience can be drawn on, conveyed or used in the context of another experience.

Sr Grant: I remember another patient who deteriorated over several weeks and died on the ward, maybe 2 years ago, who had similar problems with pain control. And ... I used my experiences from that time to apply to Hugh for strategies for helping him. (Int. 7-2: 10)

Experiences which are drawn upon may be concrete situations, complete with their inherent nuances and feelings. They may, however, also be just a word, or impression, or scene.

Experiences in the Sisters' lives outside of the work situation contribute to the meanings revealed in situations with patients and on the ward. Sr Aitkin reappraises some of her own practices, including mouth care and anticipating patients' pain, on the basis of her own experience of being a surgical patient (Int. 1-1: 24–28). The Sisters' use of their experiences echoes the research in which nurses who are parents can more ably solve the problem of a crying infant (Holden & Klingner 1988), and nurses who have suffered pain better understand the pain experience (Holm et al 1989).

As mentioned in a previous section, the Sisters are attuned to meanings in all of their experiences. This enables them to draw upon all sorts of experiences. Sr Baxter talks about growing up within a sensitive family with a Granny who 'had a great understanding of people' (Int. 2-3: 12). She says of her own understanding of people:

Sr Baxter: [. . .] . . . . . it comes from experience with people, not necessarily people in nursing. But in any experience you've had with people outside you can pick up a lot. (Int. 2-3: 11)

For the Sisters, the experience which they draw upon for practice is not confined to specific, discrete situations, nor is it confined to nursing. Sr Hanna puts it nicely when she says, '. . . my whole experience is my life . . .' and '. . . just life is your experience' (Int. 8-3: 39).

With experience comes confidence

While the Sisters have confidence which stems from their experience, they are not always confident in new positions, or in untried situations. Sr Inglis tells about experiencing her first year as a ward sister.

Sr Inglis: [It was a v]ery traumatic year for me. Because I feel that I was as good a night sister as I could be. I tried to give support and the best care a night sister can give. And I had all that stripped away in the first year I came here. I really had to re-challenge myself as a person. I found that I wasn't as good a nurse as I thought I was. I wasn't as

experienced as I thought I was. I didn't learn as quickly as I thought I was going to. And I didn't accept the change from a small hospital to a big one. So many things happened to me in that first year and it took me time to find my feet again. (Int. 9-3: 13)

In a new role, the Sister loses her feet; she does not know her way. It is only with time that she 'finds her feet', and becomes sure of her footing. The amount of time it takes to become confident varies considerably. It is almost a year before Sr Inglis feels 'home and dry' as a ward sister. On the other hand, Sr Jarvis gains confidence in her assessment of bladder clots during the course of a shift, although with time and subsequent experiences, her confidence deepens. It is not unusual for the Sisters to feel confident about some aspects of a situation and not as confident about others. They talked about coming to feel 'at home' in situations only when they were confident that they could handle the unexpected as well as what was routine.

Through experiences in practice, the Sisters come to have confidence in their own perceptions and practice. They trust their knowledge, and from this basis, act more flexibly, more confidently and with authority.

Sr Baxter: [W]ith experience comes confidence. As you're a bit more assured of what you're exactly doing and what you're doing [it] with it becomes easier . . . (Int. 2-3: 30)

Confidence as an outgrowth of experience leads the Sisters to notice and act differently. Sr Ellis' sureness of knowledge comes into how she acts as a safety net when a nurse errs in changing a tracheostomy tube.

Sr Ellis: [. . .] But, of course having changed lots of tracheostomy tubes I'm able to be more confident and to maybe press harder than they would . . . (Int. 5-1: 17)

When the replacement tracheostomy tube would not go in with a gentle push and the staff nurse was panic-stricken, Sr Ellis knew just what pressure and placement of the tube would work to get it in. Having the 'confidence of experience' (Int. 5-3: 26), the Sister understands the potential and limitations of the situation and understands her own capabilities to act. Being confident makes it easier to cope with unforeseen changes. Being able to successfully handle traumatic 'first' experiences is a great boost to confidence, as Sr Jarvis finds when she correctly assesses the bladder clot.

The Sisters use their feelings of confidence as a gauge of their experience, particularly in situations where there have been imperceptible changes over time. After a rocky beginning, Sr Inglis knows she is 'home and dry' as a new ward sister when she feels confident in her experience.

Sr Inglis: [. . .] [T]here was always apprehension coming on duty. And then one day I was no longer apprehensive and I realized that I was home. (Int. 9-3: 10)

Confidence also accompanies understanding one's own limitations in the job. Sr Grant's confidence allows her to acknowledge that not all problems can be solved; some can only be contained (W7D4: 21). Through the self-understanding and the confidence which comes with experience, the Sisters recognize their own strengths and limitations. This may be one of the reasons why several of the Sisters say they get more satisfaction from nursing now than they did when they were students. Their experience and confidence allows them to get 'closer to the patients' and 'get more out of nursing'. When the Sisters are confident, they feel at home in their jobs and in their ward situations. They have the comfort of dwelling in the situations they encounter.

Confidence changes understanding

Over time, the understanding of similar experiences changes. What was major, becomes minor; what was challenging and uncommon becomes commonplace and routine. The Sisters' confidence in their own abilities, know-how and practices, and their confident understanding of the patients and the medical and ward practices, all contribute to such a change.

To Sr Fraser, the care of a complex laryngectomy patient which was once new and challenging, is now 'routine' (Int. 6-3: 29). She knows what to do and what to expect. Sr Grant describes 2 days,

which I found as an observer to be complex and thought-provoking, as 'fairly typical' and '. . . not notable, in any way, really' (Int. 7-3: 1). They are routine for her. The days are:

Sr Grant: Fairly typical of, of life here.
M.M.:   Can you think of what makes them typical?
Sr Grant: Ah . . . similar sorts of problems. Problems that that have cropped up before, the same frustrations. Just the repetition of a pattern. (Int. 7-3: 2)

With experience, the Sisters' repertoire of skills and familiar situations increases. They see patterns in their own experiences and in their work situations. More of their knowledge becomes taken-for-granted, and different aspects of situations become salient. Their experiences of similar situations change.

As many patients undergo similar surgical procedures on the wards, the Sisters find that many situations become routine over time. They have few opportunities to say, 'Oh I've not come across that before. Now what are we going to do about it' (Int. 10-3: 21). Usually, the routine nature of the surgery is overshadowed by the Sister's attention to the individual concerns of the people undergoing the procedures, and by the complexities of keeping the ward working in ever changing circumstances. Sometimes, however, the routine nature of the work is problematic. In Chapter 7, I discuss some ways in which the Sisters keep themselves noticing and attuned to their experiences in routine situations so that they keep their practice in question and do not become falsely confident.

Confidence, then, is one of the indicators of the movement of experience. Confidence indicates a movement in understanding about oneself and one's capabilities. Confidence not only comes out of experience, it also helps the Sisters to be open to new experience. Confident in their abilities to see, hear and remember, the Sisters extend the range of what they notice; confident in their interpretations of situations, the Sisters try out new ways of interacting, and act with sureness; confident in themselves, the Sisters are not afraid to take risks and practise more flexibly. As we shall see in the following chapters, confidence features in the Sisters' practice and learning.

SUMMARY

Experience, I have argued, is more complex than it is usually portrayed in the research literature. Particularly in the experiential learning literature, experience is considered to be an entity which contains sense data; other research, including some phenomenological studies, is primarily concerned with the meanings contained within experience. In contrast to the depiction of experience as a static, spatial entity from which meanings or data can be extracted, the examination of the Sisters' accounts and practices has revealed experience to be complex, continually changing and elusive. The Sisters' everyday experience has been seen to be inextricably bound with their ongoing, moment-by-moment practices.

On close examination of the interviews and field notes, two ways of understanding experience have emerged. Experience has been found to be a resource or entity, something which the person has or could gain. However, more importantly perhaps, it also has been found to be an ongoing process — a process of experiencing. These two senses of experience have not been found to be separate. Rather, they are in continual interplay, with the experience in the sense of a resource growing out of, informing and being changed by the process of experiencing.

Experience takes a variety of forms in the Sisters' accounts and practices; I have depicted the range of forms by delineating three: 'watershed', 'resonant' and 'bits and bobs'.

'Watershed experiences' are highly memorable, often first-time instances which are emotionally charged, specifically meaningful for the Sister and vividly told. They are specific situations in which the Sisters' understanding is considerably altered. They are similar to Benner's (1984, 1994) paradigm cases.

'Resonant experiences' are less emotionally charged and often take place over a longer period of time. Patients who are memorable in specific contexts are often the subject. These experiences also may be the result of an accumulation of taken-for-granted experiences in which a gradual change in self-understanding is realized. Typically, the narrative form of 'resonant experiences' is less coherent; they need prompting to be recalled.

'Bits and bobs', forming by far the majority of experiences, happen all the time and are taken-for-granted. They concern the Sisters' ongoing practising, are often forgotten soon afterwards or are not considered to be important enough to talk about. As 'bits and bobs' experiences may be kinesic experience, they may remain tacit and unspoken. They rarely come into the interviews and only then as a result of direct questioning.

When the interplay of experiences and experiencing was examined, experience was found to be grounded in concrete activities in time and place. The Sisters experience their practice within a temporal situation, an historical situation. As the situation changes, so does their experience. In experience there is a continual interplay between the past and present, with a sense of expectation towards the future. There is a movement in understanding. In addition to the negation of previous understanding, in everyday taken-for-granted situations, understanding is extended, enriched and confirmed.

Experience happens on a ground of meaning in which situations and people matter to the Sisters. The Sisters are attuned, and pick up the meanings inherent in practice situations and in experiences outwith the practice situation. Their stance of concern and involvement in the situation contributes to the ways in which they pick up on meanings. Further experiences cast new light on old situations, bringing forth hitherto unidentified meanings. Experience is not compartmentalized by the Sisters; they draw on experience gained both outside and inside nursing. Confidence plays a special role. It seems to be one of the significant outgrowths of experience and features in the Sisters' ability to bring their experience into practice situations.

Experience can perhaps best be depicted as movement: a process which is interlinked with ongoing practising; an interplay between the experiences which the Sisters already have and the ongoing process of experiencing. In experiencing there is movement: in time, and in understanding of both practice and oneself.

The problem in linking the interview and observational material to the notion of experience has already been raised, but such material is perhaps the best we can expect to gather on such an ephemeral phenomenon. Although experience is a personal, individual matter, it is also constituted in a social world and its public form is in the Sisters' practices. In the next chapter, I describe what the Sisters are doing in their everyday nursing practice. The central focus of their practice is helping the individual patient towards recovery, but in order to do that they make the ward work for all the patients. This focus in practice, on the individual patient in the context of the ward, parallels the Sisters' expression of their experience. They express a deep understanding of individuals in complex, and often difficult, situations.

Notes

[1] In a more recent study, Benner (1991, Benner et al 1992) attends more directly to learning and to the role of narrative in learning.

[2] All nurse and patient names are pseudonyms.

[3] In phenomenology, it is common to excavate the ground and grounding of a phenomenon in order more clearly to see and understand the phenomenon.

[4] In *The Primacy of Caring*, Benner refines her use of experience, particularly with regard to life experience. 'Experience does not mean simply a passage through time, it means the way in which one is changed, for better or for worse, by what happens to one. Life experience changes meanings, understanding, and skills' (Benner & Wrubel 1989 p 104).

5

Surgical nursing practice

INTRODUCTION

Sr Jarvis: [. . . .] One thing I like about Surgical Unit is the fact that you bring patients in and you make them unwell and you make them better again. And that's always been something I think of as NURSING. We make these people unwell and then it's up to us to make them better again. (Int. 10-1: 15)

Patients play a pivotal role in the understanding of experience which emerges through an examination of the Sisters' everyday practice. Patients are the reason the Sisters practise nursing; they provide the situations within which the Sisters experience nursing. In the last chapter we saw something of the nature of the Sisters' experience and how it is linked to everyday practice. Clearly, experience consists of more than just isolated events: it is intertwined with ongoing, moment-by-moment, everyday practice.

This chapter, then, is concerned with the Sisters' everyday nursing practice. The Sisters' primary goal is to help surgical patients towards recovery[1]. However, nursing practice in a ward is a collective endeavour. It is led by the Ward Sister who determines the work to be done, organizes the nurses to provide care to patients and ensures that the work is undertaken to a particular standard. In order to help individual patients towards recovery, the Ward Sisters must make the ward work for all.

The organization of the discussion in this chapter reflects the Sisters' experiences of the patients and the ward. In their accounts of experiences with patients, the Sisters usually set situations or concerns within the framework of the patients' stay on the ward. This frame is reflected in daily practices: at the change of shift handover reports, the nurses tell about the patients in relation to their stay. In keeping with this, the discussion about helping individual patients towards recovery is broadly structured around familiar landmarks in the patients' stay. In contrast, the discussion of the Sisters' practices, which make the ward work, is structured around the workflow of a single shift. This structure parallels the Sisters' experiences of the work of the ward which is captured in the phrase, commonly expressed by them, 'Today's another day'. Their practices and experiences are complex. Contributing to this complexity is their focus on the care of each patient while making the ward work for all of the patients. Also contributing are the divergent temporal experiences of the patients through their stay, and the work of the ward through the day.

The richness of the material in the interviews and field notes has provided a marvellous resource with which to create a vivid tapestry of the Sisters' practices. The focus of the book, however, is every-day experience, and a fuller depiction of the Sisters' practices must remain secondary to this. Therefore, in the discussion which follows, I hope to provide a glimpse of the Sisters' everyday practice and experience with patients in the ward. While only a glimpse, it will provide a context for the discussions about the process of practising and experiencing practice in the next chapters.

HELPING PATIENTS TOWARDS RECOVERY

The Sisters' practices are directly and indirectly geared towards helping patients who are admitted to the surgical wards to prepare for surgery and to recover from it. What is striking about their practices is how active and complex they are. This perspective is missing from the research literature on recovery from surgery, perhaps because in most of these studies, the discussion concentrates on the patients' experience of recovery (cf. Webb 1984, 1986, Baker 1989) and more commonly, on the patients' recovery process and specific interventions which influence it, such as information-giving, pain relief and exercise (cf. Hayward 1975, Wilson-Barnett & Fordham 1982, Johnson 1984, Devine 1992).

Wilson-Barnett (1988) suggests that these studies as a whole show that the type of intervention a nurse provides is 'often a mixture of psychological support, physical coping skills, health education and practical advice'. I would argue, however, that the studies portray the nurse as peripheral to the patients' recovery. They show the patient recovering from surgery with minimal nursing input, and with few exceptions, the input appears mechanistic. In many studies, the nurse is virtually invisible. However, when the Sisters' experience is examined directly, a different view emerges. With their extensive repertoire of complex practices, the Sisters are seen to actively help patients through their surgical admission.

The patients in surgical wards

Surgeons admit people to surgical wards because they are seen to have a problem which might benefit from surgical treatment. There are several routes to admission. The route taken has implications for the patients' needs, expectations and understanding about hospitalization and care, and in turn, for the Sisters' practices.

Patients may be admitted as 'emergency admissions' on an 'external waiting' day or night from Accident and Emergency or from another ward on an 'internal waiting' day. Patients also may be admitted to the ward from the outpatient clinic. These patients have been seen by the registrar or consultant and urgently need hospital-ization. Patients in these two groups sometimes have complex problems which need to be diagnosed and 'sorted out' or treated in hospital before surgical treatment is planned.

Planned admissions, the third route, come from the consultants' waiting lists; patients are given a specific time and day to come in. Their course of treatment is more predictable and the patients are somewhat prepared for hospitalization. The final route of admission is through temporary transfer. Patients come from another surgical ward as 'boarders' when the other ward is over-flowing or closing for the weekend or holidays.

In the study wards, the decision to admit and discharge or transfer patients is always a medical decision but one which nurses influence. The nurses on a ward care for all patients on that ward as well as for patients who are attached to the ward on an emergency or outpatient basis. They are also responsible for the discharge arrangements for patients who may be 'boarded out' to other wards.

'Presenting yourself': creating the possibility for patients to engage in a trusting relationship

The patients' arrival on the ward signals the beginning of their stay and the beginning of their relationship with the ward staff. The Sisters recognize this as an important time, a time of first impressions, when patients do or don't begin to feel comfortable in the ward and to have confidence and trust in the nurses. The patients' experience during this time can set the tone for their entire hospital stay. The Sisters aim to make the patients' stay on the ward, a 'smooth passage' from the time of their admission to the time of their discharge.

All of the Sisters ensure that new patients coming into the ward are acknowledged when they arrive, even though they might have to wait before being attended to. They recognize the vulnerability of patients at this time and the importance of first impressions.

Sr Ellis: [. . .] You see them all sitting there, and they stare and they watch every movement that you make. And if they're seeing someone clomping up and down the corridor or [. . .] shouting, you can imagine what must be going through their minds: 'Are these people going to be looking after me?' (Int. 5-1: 21)

The Sisters take particular care to introduce themselves to new patients.

Sr Grant: I now see that there are times that are particularly important when you present yourself. And one of them is the first 30 seconds of your contact with the patient. (Int. 7-3: 17)

In presenting themselves, the Sisters are present with the patient. They tell the patient who they are and confirm the patient's name. Presenting 'yourself' characterizes the nature of the relationship which the Sisters seek to develop — personal, yet purposeful; a relationship between individuals. During such encounters, the Sisters acknowledge both the patients and their concerns. Because of conflicting demands on their time the Sisters

have developed techniques which help them to engage the patients in a relationship in a very short period of time.

0955 — Sr Inglis [. . .] goes to take some pillows to the left cubicle. Mr Ball is in there, having just come in with his wife. He says he is nervous. She tells him that if he wasn't nervous she would be surprised. She jokes with him, 'I won't bite and I don't scratch' and then she says that his wife could stay, that they were very busy and it would be a while before a nurse [comes] to admit him. (W9D4: 11)
Sr Inglis describes her approach:
Sr Inglis: You see I've got a little knack. And I'm not sure if it's good or not. I can pull somebody's leg, which means that I'm paying attention to them and I'm aware of them but it saves me from giving them any more time. To make him feel just that little bit of home, a quick joke. [. . .] When I explained I didn't have a nurse. I didn't want him dismissed and him sitting there thinking, 'My God!'. So a quick joke and somehow it might just be peculiar to British people. I don't know cause we don't nurse many foreign people. It does seem to work with British people. (Int. 9-1: 18)

The Sisters, each in their own way, manage the tension between taking time for one patient and attending to all. They have developed practices which allow them to give what they can at the time to patients, to acknowledge them and their concerns, thus making them feel welcome, and beginning to establish a rapport. These are not just rote practices. Neither is it 'emotional labour' designed to induce or suppress feeling to sustain an outward countenance which produces the proper state of mind in others (Hochschild 1983). The Sisters become engaged with the patients. Their practices reflect their understanding that they are relating to patients as individual people (just as they themselves are individual), '. . . but *we're* individuals' (Int. 9-2: 31). In questioning her practice, Sr Inglis points to a flexibility of approach. In common with other Sisters, she acknowledges that what works for one patient may not work for others.

Establishing a climate of reciprocal trust (Thorne & Robinson 1988) at the time of admission is critical with patients who have had problems in previous admissions or who may have difficulty coping with the institutional milieu of the hospital. For example, Sr Hanna helps to make 'a smoother passage' for Linda, a 33-year-old drug abuser, who is admitted for a laparoscopy and sterilization.

Sr Hanna knows Linda from previous admissions, the most recent of which, a week earlier, was marked by difficulty and mistrust, starting with an altercation with the nurse who admitted her and culminating with Linda effecting her own discharge. When she arrives this time, Sr Hanna greets her at the door and admits her herself. During the admission process, Linda expresses concerns that her medications are not all written up in a familiar way[2]. Sr Hanna explains the many medications, but then says, 'But we will get these written up right' (W8D2-1: 20). She goes directly to the Resident:

She asks him to write the meds up, the AZT and DF118, 'in a more particular way as she expects it to be, with the exact times'. He says, 'That's fine' and strikes out the two orders and writes them differently. (W8D2-1: 20)

By smoothly arranging the change in the medication order and being present in a calm and cheering way, Sr Hanna creates a non-threatening atmosphere for Linda. The effect on Linda is noticeable.

(Sr Hanna's report to the late staff) 'Linda [. . .] is like a different person this time :: She is most cooperative :: She is not keeping a constant record of our conversations. :: You would hardly recognize her as the same person.' (W8D2-2: 14)

Hearing and attending to patients' particular concerns at this time, creates a climate of trust and creates possibilities for a 'smooth passage' in hospital. When the Sisters present themselves, they begin to engage the patient in a relationship which can positively influence the patient's stay on the ward.

Helping people to prepare for surgery

In the preoperative period, the Sisters coordinate the various diagnostic and physical preparations for patients, tailoring them as needed to individuals. Adjusting preparations to suit the person ranges from negotiating with the anaesthetist to provide a nasogastric tube in theatre for a patient who is particularly anxious (W9D4: 10), to ensuring that the Registrar marks the spot for an ileostomy stoma for a young man when he is wearing his usual trousers (W9D4: 7). Preoperatively, the

Sisters play a major part in confirming, correcting and extending the patients' understanding of what is likely to happen during surgery and afterwards. When patients require emergency or unexpected surgery, this preparation can be complex. The Sister needs to assess and address the patient's specific needs for preparation, including information, usually in a fairly short period of time. The following extended example illustrates an intensive, complex, but not unusual process.

Usually patients with cancer of the larynx are diagnosed and 'worked up' in the outpatient clinic and the ear, nose and throat ward over a 2-week period prior to laryngectomy. Mr Peet, a 73-year-old man who comes into the ward on a Tuesday directly from being seen in clinic, has less than 2 days to prepare. On Wednesday, Mr Peet has a direct laryngoscopy and a large tumour is seen, which is punctured on examination and an emergency tracheostomy undertaken. It is Thursday and a 4-day holiday weekend begins on Friday. Two hours before the following conversation takes place, the Registrar discusses the surgery, scheduled for Friday, with Mr Peet. As Sr Ellis goes into the room, Mr Peet is sitting up in his bed, with a nebulizer covering his tracheostomy.

Sr Ellis goes in to see Mr Peet and Nurse Neale [a student nurse who is 'specialling' Mr Peet] :: They are talking for a bit, and he is looking pretty agitated :: Sr Ellis says something about him having the operation tomorrow and he writes 'I don't want it' :: He looks frightened and says [mouthing as he can't speak], 'No, no, no, I don't want it.' [. . .]
Sr Ellis: 'They think it is the best thing for you.' She continues but the conversation doesn't seem to be going anywhere.
Nurse Neale is on one side of the bed and Sr Ellis is on the other. Sr Ellis starts squatting down beside the bed so she is below him, but as he starts to protest about the operation, she gets closer to him, at eye level. As he protests a bit more, she backs away a bit, but she says softly 'I think you're scared. I think that's it'.
Then all of a sudden, it is as though there is an opening and she takes it :: She does most of the talking and he listens, looking ever more intently at her face as she talks, as though he is mesmerized, but taking it in :: She is looking directly at him the whole time.
Sr Ellis: 'She's a "bossy boots" type doctor :: She's new :::: She's been upstairs :: but she's good :: So when they're new, they try to :: :: :::
'Can I just go back to the beginning and go over it

with you? :: My name is Fiona :: You've got cancer in your voice box :: That's making it hard to breathe :: [. . .] And I get quite breathless so I know a bit of what you're feeling when you're out of breath :: It gives you quite a fright :: ::
'So what happened yesterday is :: There's a growth on your voice box :: right where the tube was :: The tumour was right there :: So they took a specimen :: . . . Some people think that once the tumour is open or cut into it spreads :: People think once it's been tampered with, you have to do something about it :: They don't know if that's true or old wives' tales ::: You think that's why they want to do it right away [he nods] 'Usually people have time to prepare :: but you don't have the time :: They think you have a good chance of success :: It's as close to a cure :: I can't guarantee there is a cure, but they wouldn't do it if they didn't think there was a good chance of success :: There's a holiday tomorrow and it would cost twice as much to the health service to have it done. I mean, we're here anyway :: The doctors, on their own time are coming in :: They wouldna do that unless they thought you had a good chance :: You'll be OK. ::
'It will be the same sort of anaesthetic as before :: You made it through that one :: There will be some stitches here [pointing to her throat and to his] and you will have this tube in [pointing to the nasogastric tube] :: This hole in your throat is temporary, but they will make a permanent one :: You will get a breathing tube which will be permanent :: You could go home with it and eat with it :: You canna eat with this tube and if you went home you couldna care for this one :: But you could go home with the other tube ::
'When the voice box is taken out a person doesn't breathe through your nose, but you're not breathing through it now :: :: and you won't be able to talk :: but you're no able to talk now :: you'll take the tube out and the hole will still be there :: It is like putting your teeth in in the morning :: There is no chance of cure or going home with this one. [referring to the tube he has in at present] You will be able to eat :: and you would get back to your normal life :: so at the moment :: this tube is in for life ::' *He's starting to look less angry and frightened and a bit more accepting.*
'Dr Smith means well :: Don't put too much into how she said it :: She says things pretty straight :: We'll be telling you lots of things :: :: Do you normally have a wee nip? [He nods] How would you like me to put some down your tube? It might help to calm your nerves a bit. [He says vigorously, 'NO'] :: The doctor will be coming in to put in your antibiotic :: your milk is due now [looking at Nurse Neale who says, 'Yes, I'll do it'] :: Now, we'll put the sides up [putting the sides of the bed up] You can grab one to get up or down :: If you have any questions at all or anything you want to ask us :: just ask :: I'll speak to your family when they come in :: Your family called, by the way, this morning :: I said you had had a good night ::' *He is looking much*

calmer by this time and has a look in his eye as though he is thankful to her. (W5D2-1: 5–6)

In this 15-minute conversation, Sr Ellis picks up that Mr Peet's protests stem from feeling frightened; she supports the doctor's decision and skill, but not her approach; she talks about the things which other people facing laryngectomy have felt frightened about and, through that process, addresses Mr Peet's fears so that he comes to understand his situation. She sets the scene for more information and preparation. This conversation is a starting point for preparations with the dietitian, the speech therapist and the physiotherapist in which Sr Ellis cues each about Mr Peet's needs.

Although the conversation as verbally recorded is like a monologue, it is a dialogue as Sr Ellis attends to Mr Peet's non-verbal cues and responds to them. She notices the fine changes in his responses and adjusts her tone, physical stance, speaking and pacing to what she finds.

In the afternoon, Sr Ellis takes the opportunity to go through the preparations again when Mr Peet's cousin visits. The nature of this conversation indicates that Mr Peet is coming to understand what is happening and to accept the need for surgery. Sr Ellis begins to mobilize Mr Peet's family to provide support through this disfiguring surgery. In the afternoon, Sr Ellis brings a patient who underwent a laryngectomy 2 weeks previously to meet Mr Peet. This is a risk since each man is still coming to terms with his new situation. However, the risk pays off, as both men indicate the following day (W5D2-2: 13).

In these conversations, Sr Ellis links what is familiar to what is unknown. She links Mr Peet's knowledge of having the temporary tube, with the tube to be put in and his knowledge of going through an anaesthetic with the anaesthetic to come. She does not minimize his concerns but uses his experiences to reduce some of his fear and anxiety. She also uses the experiences of others, in discussion and in person, to make the unfamiliar and frightening a little less so for both Mr Peet and his family. As much as she can, Sr Ellis arranges to have the time she needs with Mr Peet, and to have others there at opportune times for him and his family. Throughout the shift, Sr Ellis stops at the door of the room to monitor the situation. As Sr Ellis handles the complex and difficult task of helping Mr Peet come to terms with his situation, while supporting Nurse Neale to give direct care, she fosters a climate of reciprocal trust and knowledgeable care.

During the preoperative period, the Sister gets to know a bit about the patient and his or her response to being in hospital. It often forms the baseline which the Sister uses for recognizing subtle changes in the person postoperatively, which indicate problems or progression in recovery. In emergency admissions, when this initial baseline is missing or the patient is in a stressed state, the Sisters have more difficulty knowing what to aim for and encourage. However, what they glean from their contacts with the patient and family preoperatively, they draw upon as they care for the patient following the operation.

'He's coming along as expected': facilitating postoperative recovery

Metaphors used by the Sisters when discussing aspects of postoperative recovery express movement towards something: a journey, as in 'he's on his way', or in the case of complications, a game or battle — 'he's back to square one' or 'he's had a setback'. When faced with problems in recovery, the patient needs to 'overcome hurdles', 'get over the hump' or 'get clear of the problems'. When the recovery journey is going well, it is described as 'smooth' or 'progressing well' or 'progressing as expected'. From their experience of many patients in similar situations, the Sisters recognize 'usual' patterns of recovery and link their understanding of a particular patient's progress to what might be expected. However, it is impossible to extract from the Sisters' practice either rules for monitoring care or discrete phases of recovery. Their actual care of individual patients reveals a much more fluid and subtle yet active process than is described in textbook treatments of postoperative care. In the patients' postoperative stay in hospital, there are some notable ways in which the Sisters help patients towards recovery.

Diligently watching

Upon the patients' return from the operating theatre, the Sisters begin a period of closely monitoring individual aspects of the patients' physical status, including pulse, blood pressure, respirations, bleeding, pain, and in many cases, fluid balance. In patients with more complex conditions, some of these physical parameters are measured mechanically. At the same time, the Sisters gather a total picture or impression of the patient in the bed, including the monitored signs and their significance. With experience, nurses become astute at picking up small changes in the patients' condition, what Benner (1984) terms 'graded qualitative distinctions'. The Sisters monitor each patient through the assigned nurses and focus selectively, 'keeping a close eye on' patients whose conditions are less stable.

In the following example, Sr Jarvis, with a first year student, diligently watches a patient newly back from surgery, picks up the 'early warning signals' (Benner 1984) of postoperative bleeding and acts on them. In contrast to the similar situation discussed in Chapter 4, where Sr Jarvis only responded once the patient was in severe pain and the bladder clot had formed, Sr Jarvis attends to more subtle signs of bleeding and acts much earlier, preventing the need for further surgery.

Sr Jarvis: [Mr Scott] was a gentleman who'd had a prostatectomy and he came back with bladder irrigation. Which was unusual because the consultant who'd operated normally uses [?] and furosemide and doesn't use irrigation. So I immediately thought that the reason for this must be that he'd had a large prostate resection. And his urine on return was really quite darkly haematuric.

So I said to the student who was looking after him that she had to be particularly careful at making sure that his irrigation always ran fully on, so that there was no chance of it clotting off. And to keep a very close eye on his urine output. That it was very haematuric, more so than we would like. His blood pressure and pulse on return were comparable with his pre-op. But I told her to make sure she would let me know if it started to fall.

About an hour later she told me that his blood pressure had dropped by about 30 mm diastolic and so I then immediately increased his IV fluids. And phoned the Resident. [. . .] His blood pressure continued to drop and his urine still remained very haematuric so we started blood transfusions. (Int. 10-2: 21–23)

Following blood transfusions, the administration of atropine and about 3 hours of penile traction, the bleeding stopped and 'everything then went according to plan' (Int. 10-2: 23).

In this situation, Sr Jarvis was alerted to the potential for bleeding because of a variation in the surgeon's usual postoperative procedure. The potential was confirmed by the quality of haematuria. 'I wasn't happy with him from the minute he came back' (Int. 10-2: 24). On the Urology Ward, the nurses recognize a range of haematuria and its significance in relation to normal progression or difficulties in recovery. Sr Jarvis includes a number of facets in assessing the patient and the significance of the clinical signs. She assesses how the patient says he feels ('he said he felt fine'), how he appears, and when that changes.

He initially looked fine [...] and just prior to the blood transfusion being started he looked to me quite pale. I noted he was a little bit clammy. (Int. 10-2: 24)

By understanding how quickly a patient's condition can change when he is bleeding, Sr Jarvis alerts the student to the importance of 'diligently watching patients from the minute they come back' (Int. 10-2: 24), and averts a more serious situation.

Recovery from the anaesthetic and the immediate effect of an operation takes from 2 to 48 hours for most patients. Barring complications, when patients pass a turning point, 'the hump', the Sisters consider them to be 'on their way to recovery'. Diligent watching continues until the Sisters sense the patients are over the hump.

'Helping patients over the hump'

Surgery interrupts both the body's physiological integrity and the patient's feeling of wholeness. The Sisters pick up the signs which indicate that patients are moving over the humps of the early stages of recovery and feeling 'themselves' again. These signs are simple, such as a change in focus of attention, interest in an event in the outside world, interest in appearance or even being ready to wear false teeth. Sometimes there is no specific sign, it is an overall sense. '[It's] a feeling that you can see [...] They just LOOK better' (Int. 2-2: 19–20).

Building on that sense of the patients' readiness to move forward, the Sisters encourage recovery in small ways. They gradually involve patients in making more decisions about their care, help people to regain normal movement, and anticipate and guide patients and their families to understand new possibilities of action.

The Sisters' encouragement may be subtle. In the immediate phase of recovering from anaesthetic and operation, they give patients choices in such things as getting dressed, having a bath, or having pain medication before eating (for newly post-op tonsillectomy patients), but do it in a voice and turn of phrase which implies no choice, 'You'll have a bath now?' Later, the Sister gives the patient a real choice, again by phrasing and her use of voice.

At this time the Sisters' approach is much like a coach (manager) who is trying to mobilize the potential of the players (Benner 1984).

When Sr Calder takes basins to a couple of men in the side ward she says, 'Fingers', and indicates that Grant and John [who had surgery on their arms] are to do their finger exercises. [She stands facing] Grant: 'Yes you can'. *She and he do it together. She has her fingers up, showing him. He can see them* 'Push, push, push!' *Slowly, with her face screwed up and looking like she is making effort too, she moves hers up as he does. He is looking at her as he does it.* 'Good!! See — you CAN do it ... It's up to you. We can't do any more. We can do the surgery :: You have to take it from here.' (W3D2: 6)

Sr Calder suggests to John that he get a bath and move his arm in it. He tries it, sceptically, and is delighted with the way in which he is able to move his arm in the water. He begins to re-learn his taken-for-granted, normal range of motion. In another situation, Sr Fraser gives tablets rather than syrup to a quinsy patient who is reluctant to swallow in order to assess his capacity for swallowing as well as to help him exercise his throat muscles (W6D4: 11). The Sisters notice the patients' potential for recovery, understand what is needed to regain normal action, and when it can occur. They help patients to recognize and re-engage their normal bodily understanding through specific exercises as well as through simple everyday activities.

Sometimes the patient loses the will for recovery, no longer seeing a purpose for recovery or a possibility of regaining health. In these situations, the Sisters talk about their active role in 'pushing' the patient or in some cases, 'battling for the patient'. The Sisters see possibilities which patients do not see and actively attempt to engage patients in seeing these possibilities for themselves.

Sr Inglis: There was an [. . .] old man who'd lost his wife this year. He admitted that he had nothing to go home for. And we had a battle to get him to Convalescent Hospital. He was a dear old soul. You could have done what you liked with him, he wouldn't have put up any effort. So you needed to instil in him, the will to live if you like. The reason for going home. [. . .]

Well he was very depressed one day and he didn't want to eat. [. . .] You could get him up out of the chair and do what you LIKED with him. [. . .] He wouldn't put up any resistance. But you knew it was just being a puppet if you like. And one day I said, 'You're miserable and depressed aren't you?' He said, 'Yes'. And I said, 'Now I know you've lost your wife. Do you feel you've nothing to go home to, nothing to live for'. And that was just it. And once we'd established that, once someone had been honest with him and said, 'Well I can understand that, but you can't throw in the towel can you?'

He'd a daughter, a son who were very loving. His daughter, [. . .] came in every single day. Brought the grandchildren in. So we had to use that as a stepping stone for him. And say, 'Come on. You know they're coming EVERY day. Don't you think you should try just a little harder? Just even today'. And that's how slowly we got him there. (Int. 9-2: 12)

Sr Inglis captures what is preventing this man from becoming reintegrated with his world and helps to harness and mobilize his will to live. Drawing on what they know of the patient preoperatively and from the patient's family, the Sisters intervene with a timing and pacing that maintains a productive tension between pushing the patient and 'going with him' in his own time. Just as Sr Ellis assesses the potential support which Mr Peet's family can give as she draws them into the preoperative preparations, so the other Sisters carefully mobilize the family to help patients towards recovery.

Bringing patients 'into the body of the kirk': promoting recovery through a place in the ward

The Sisters use the space in their wards to promote patients' physical recovery and to help patients re-engage in a social milieu. Patients are placed in particular beds to facilitate their observation and care by the nurses, to promote their socializing with other patients, for ease of walking to the toilet, for control of infection, and for other reasons. On the Nightingale wards, ill patients are usually at the 'head' of the ward, near the nursing station for ease of observation and attention. As they recover, patients are moved farther 'down' the ward, or 'out' into a side ward. Sr Aitkin discusses her plans to move Mrs Jones, a 72-year-old woman with an above-the-knee amputation, who is reluctant to take an interest in her food and is fearful of going to the Rehabilitation Hospital.

'[I think we will] bring her into the 'body of the kirk' for a couple of reasons . . . So she is not so near the nursing station :: She might feel not quite so sick. When they're down this way, they talk more. She'll see others in situations like her own. Mrs Harper [a lady with an above-the-knee amputation] will talk with her. She will see how well Mrs Harper is doing. Mrs Harper has been to Rehabilitation Hospital and Mrs Jones will be going there tomorrow. She will see that Mrs Harper has to have another leg off, so she won't feel so sorry for herself. She will see the leg Mrs Harper has. It will give Mrs Harper something to do to keep her mind off her own problems, and off thinking about her own operation'. (W1D3: 1)

The Sisters recognize the support and example which other patients provide and set up situations for this to happen. They recognize the meaning of placement in the ward for the patients and their families and incorporate this into their care. After clearing it with their bacteriologist, Sr Inglis brings a patient onto the ward who has a severe *Clostridium Welchii* (gas gangrene) infection and has been nursed in the cubicle for 10 days. The move has a marked effect on his depression. 'Slowly over that period he began to take notice and perked up' (Int. 9-2: 5). It was also a good prognostic sign for his wife. 'I think she felt a sense of relief somehow that maybe he was off the danger list by doing that' (Int. 9-2: 6).

The Sisters understand the meanings which being in certain places have for patients and their families at various times in the recovery process. A place in the ward can both indicate and promote recovery. Being in certain places is also of particular importance as patients become ready for discharge, as we shall see shortly.

'Getting it right for you': addressing common problems individually

Although postoperative pain and wounds have been the focus of much nursing research, the meaning of pain and wounds for patients is not readily discernible in much of the literature (cf. Seers 1987, Fordham 1988, Brunner & Suddarth 1992, Closs 1992, Alexander et al 1994). This would be noteworthy in itself given the self-evident importance of understanding pain and wounds from the perspective of the patient. It takes on added significance here, as will become apparent, since the meaning of pain and wounds for individual patients and their recovery figures highly in the Sisters' practices of pain control and wound care.

In familiar situations, the Sisters use the amount of pain a patient is experiencing as an indicator of recovery. A certain amount of pain can be expected at some points; if the patient experiences more, it indicates actual or potential problems, requiring nursing action. Sr Aitkin persists in getting the Resident to bi-valve a cast on Mrs Harper 2 hours after amputation, on the basis of the patient's complaints of pain which are out of step with the amount of pain medication she had received. The bi-valving releases the pressure from a slipped drain and poorly applied dressing. Sr Aitkin acted on intuition: 'I've known her for a long time ... She had pain' (W1D5: 11).

Understanding the meaning of pain is often difficult, particularly when the Sister does not know the patient's normal response to pain, or

when the operation is a new or unfamiliar one. The Sisters talk about trying to understand whether the pain might be 'in the operation', or whether it is 'in the patient' (W8D2-1: 10). That is, they try to understand the nature of pain that can be expected: including how much pain, where it is located, what kind of pain it is, what it feels like and when it occurs.

The Sisters want the patients' pain to be controlled in a way that suits the patient. On one ward, where many patients have chronic pain and are on large doses of morphine, the consultant joked, 'Good — now Sister's back all the patients will be awake' (W1D1: 11). The Sisters fine tune the amounts of medication, and administration times so that patients are awake, able to move as they need to and ready for meals at mealtimes. The Sisters aim for an optimal analgesic cover, so patients are neither over nor undermedicated. Methods such as pain charts are sometimes used to help patients communicate clearly with the nurses about intractable pain so that their medication can be adjusted accordingly.

The Sisters recognize that giving analgesia in an anticipatory way might not be best for everyone in all situations. The goal is to 'keep on top' of the pain in an appropriate way. They discriminate between the need for more analgesia and the need for another approach. When a nervous first-year student says to Sr Hanna that the woman to whom she was giving her first day post-op bath needs more analgesia, Sr Hanna considers the request in its context. She looks at the patient, confirms that her analgesia should still be covering her, talks calmly to both the student and the patient, telling the patient what the student will be doing and suggests that the bath should help to alleviate the pain. When the patient asks what she could do to relax, Sr Hanna suggests, smiling, 'Talk about anything but your operation. Nurse, keep her away from that topic'. With that, both student and patient appear less anxious; the student proceeds with the bath and the patient declines pain medication until 2 hours later (W8D2-1: 7).

Characteristically, the Sisters remain attuned to the importance and significance to the patient of what is routine to the nurse. Removing sutures is a good example. As Sr Dunn takes sutures out of Mr Law's long thoracotomy wound, she attends to his anxiety, asks whether he has experienced this before, gives him an idea as to how long it will take, distracts him by asking about his plans for going home and works quickly. She repeatedly glances at his face during the procedure and asks him whether he has pain when she is about half way through (about 45 seconds into the procedure). While she is cleaning the wound she says, 'That's all out. The wound looks fine. You can have plenty of showers on it. It's well healed'. Anticipating what he might be thinking, she states it. 'People don't believe it that you can go home like this 7 days after a big operation like this.' Mr Law nods and looks relieved (W4D2-1: 3). By giving him specifics about what she is doing, and in her timing and sureness of touch she completes a very routine procedure in a way that acknowledges its uniqueness for that patient. Throughout the process, she is attuned to how the patient is responding to the procedure, and modifies her movements accordingly.

The Sisters have become skilled in adapting wound dressing materials to individual patients and their wounds. The Sisters develop their technique uniquely with each patient in response to his or her specific needs.

Sr Grant: Well the technique for doing the dressing, for instance ... how to get the patient to hold his legs so that it's most comfortable.

It's interesting. If you do the dressing one day, the patient says, 'Now Mary did this and Mary did that and if you do this it's easier'. It's not generally something that's written down because it's too inconsequential. It's just something that has developed between the patient and the nurse that usually does that dressing. (Int. 7-2: 16)

Rather than being inconsequential, these techniques could be considered skilled practices, tailored to the needs of individual patients, which develop through shared experiences of patients and nurses. When patients have repeated dressing or tube changes, this practised skill, sureness of touch and timing is critical. It has considerable impact on the patients' confidence, pain and hope.

The Ward Sisters routinely monitor slow-to-heal or chronic wounds for changes, providing continuity for the patients, their relatives, other nurses and the doctors. They do not merely observe the physical changes in the wound. The Sisters come to understand the meaning of what the wound smells like and looks like and feels like for the patient and family. They recognize the importance of this wound and find out how the patient and the family are coping. The wound is not merely 'a disruption of the integrity and function of tissues in the body' (Wilson-Barnett & Batehup 1988), but has meaning to the person and the family. Indeed, for some patients, the wound can become the centre of their existence. The Sisters incorporate their understanding of such meaning into their caring practices.

Keeping patients, families and health workers in synchrony

Sometimes during a patient's hospitalization the expectations, goals and understandings among patients, their families, doctors and nurses are in conflict or get out of step. Nurses and doctors can get out of synchrony about the plans for the patient's care. This occurance, a commonplace one, will be discussed under 'Making the ward work'. Less frequently but equally important families of patients can get out of synchrony with the doctors and nurses about the patient's problems and how health care workers are addressing them.

When the patient's prognosis is clear and optimistic, keeping the family up to date is straightforward. When the prognosis is changing or is not good (or both), the task is more difficult. For staff and families the notion of just how quickly change can be expected to occur, differs. 'Things sometimes happen too fast for families or happen too slowly' (Int. 7-2: 3). This is well illustrated in the situation of Mr Green, a man who had an amputation and subsequently suffered a stroke, an infarct and an embolus in the other leg. After the initial amputation, the nurses and the family discussed 'the likely course of events after his operation'.

Sr Grant: Then all these insults occurred. And that no longer became an appropriate plan at all. And yet family clung on to this, this plan. And his wife said to me about 2 days after his stroke, 'You said that on his third, fourth day he would be out of bed. Why is he not out of bed?' I said, 'Well things have changed and he's no longer able to support his weight. If we sat him in a chair he couldn't support his upper half. He'd just flop over. He's much more comfortable in bed'. 'What is the physiotherapist doing with him? You said that he would be given exercises to encourage him to straighten his knee and it's not happening. Why is that?' So there was no grasp that things had changed.

And it was . . . quite difficult to be quite open with them and yet not make them lose all their hope. (Int. 7-2: 4)

To get the family in synchrony the Sister has to find a balance, instilling and maintaining hope for recovery, yet not leading them towards unrealistic expectations. She helps the family towards a reasonable outlook for this patient, so they can help him in a new, but realistic, way.

In a similar situation, Sr Grant shows the family of a man who has suffered a stroke how they can best help when they come to visit.

Sr Grant: [H]e showed neglect of his left-hand side and he had a hemiopia and wouldn't attend to you at all if you stood on his left. And yet they came in and they'd sit on his left hand side and speak to him and when he didn't respond they started to raise their voices and shout as though he just wasn't hearing. (Int. 7-1: 15)

Sr Grant repeatedly explains to the patient's wife and daughter where to stand so he can perceive them, to no avail. However, a granddaughter is more perceptive and helps her grandmother to understand.

Sr Grant: 'Look what happens when I come round here. Granddad looks at me and will answer me. But if I go round here he just ignores me.' So she did it for me. (Int. 7-1: 17)

Keeping the family in synchrony includes recognizing the family's strengths and weaknesses and working with them to help the patient towards recovery or towards a peaceful death. One of the most difficult aspects of keeping the family in synchrony when the patient's prognosis is not good is 'striking a balance between being dreadfully pessimistic with [them] and being hopelessly unrealistic' (Int. 7-1: 17). Working to strike the balance implies an appreciation of the meaning of the illness experience for the patient and family, as well as understanding the possibilities inherent in the situation.

Being ready to go: helping patients to prepare for discharge

On the study wards, patients are discharged when their medical condition warrants it, and when the Ward Sisters think they are ready to go. Being ready implies more than just physical readiness. The patient must feel ready, confident enough in themselves that they will be able to manage. However, they should not be kept longer, so they 'lose the impetus to really get back to independent living' (Int. 7-3: 3). The Sisters have a clear understanding of what they can offer the patients in the ward, and what has to be offered elsewhere. Although pressure on beds means they sometimes feel that they discharge patients too soon, without sure supports at home, they practise from a sense of timing about the safe limits for discharge.

One way in which the Sisters help patients to become ready for discharge is to 'plant seeds', suggesting to the patient when he may be going home before the actual time or day of discharge. On hearing it stated, many patients turn the possibility over in their mind, begin to make arrangements and are feeling ready to go when they are discharged. Planting seeds is not only a matter of telling people what they might expect. It includes helping them experience, in a time-limited and safe way, that they can manage outside the hospital. The Sisters arrange for some patients to go home for the weekend, 'to find their feet in the outside world' (Int. 1-1: 6).

In the following example, Sr Aitkin helps a young woman with a new ileostomy get out into normal society and re-discover her self confidence.

Sr Aitkin: [. . .] We had a pub near the hospital. [. . .] [Betty] was a young girl needing to get back into society but was a little apprehensive about going out. And I said would you like to go out for a drink and she thought this was quite good but, 'Oh I can't!' she said. 'I- I- I've got nothing to wear.' And I said, 'We'll get your Mum to bring some clothes in'. And the interesting thing was that a pair of jeans [. . .] came in.

She spent all day doing her hair. She was a very pretty girl. [. . .]

And we went across to this pub and she had these very tight jeans on and we could not see her ileostomy bag. She couldn't believe that she could be dressed and people didn't know that she had an ileostomy. And she said, 'Dad gave me some money to get you a drink'. I said, 'Fine, I'll have a such and such'. And she said, 'But you go up to the bar and get it'. 'No no,' I said, 'You're treating me'. I said, 'You go up to the bar'. But she said, 'They'll all know'. And I said, 'What do you mean they'll all know?' She said, 'That I've got a bag on'. And I said, 'Why not go, you can't see it'. She said, 'I know, I know but I'm still, you know'. I wouldn't go and get the drink and I said, 'They're all going to look at you 'cause you're a very pretty girl,' I said, 'Not because of your ileostomy bag'.

And she went up to the bar, she bought the drinks and that was fine. She was so thrilled with herself that she'd actually achieved a small hurdle by going up. But nobody was aware that she had an ileostomy at all. And I felt that we'd done quite well there because she'd treated me to a drink. She was able to talk about other things. We didn't talk about hospital all night at all. (Int. 1-1: 5–6)

Going to the pub allows Betty to try a normal social situation with support from someone she knows and trusts. Betty has had time to prepare herself and the tight jeans indicate a readiness, which Sr Aitkin picks up on, pushing her to go to the bar to get the drinks. Through such ventures as this one, the Sisters help patients who have undergone major changes to regain confidence in themselves before being discharged from hospital. They make what was once familiar but is now strange, familiar and normal again.

This interplay between patients' physical recovery and their feeling of readiness to go home is assessed and promoted in different ways. Following ear surgery, on the day before discharge, the patients' first hair wash is done by a staff nurse or sister. Sr Fraser uses this opportunity to assess how the patient is, how the wound is healing, and to give information about how to care for the wound and what to expect at home (W6D2: 15).

Through practices such as these, the Sisters help patients in their passage through the ward. The practices which I have described thus far may seem, nonetheless, somewhat devoid of background. The focus has been on the Sisters and the patients, with little account taken of what else is going on at the time. Although in the everyday practice of the Sisters, the patient and the Sister are never isolated from the ongoing stream of the ward, such a focus is not out of place. When the Sisters are with individual patients, their concentration is centred on those patients. (Indeed, they recognize this themselves (Int. 4-2: 47).) However, the only way in which they can fully gear care to individual patients, and give patients concentrated attention while ensuring the care for all, is through their practices of making the ward work.

MAKING THE WARD WORK

In charge of a ward of 20 to 36 beds,[3] the Ward Sisters are responsible for:

1. Ensuring the provision of a high standard of care to patients.
2. Managing the staff and material resources of the ward.
3. Contributing to the education of students and new staff (Lewis 1990, Fitzpatrick et al 1992).

They are the coordinators and decision-makers at the centre of a complex, ever-changing network of communications, people and services (Runciman 1983). They make their wards work in a way which enables them to achieve their goal of helping individual patients towards recovery (or to die peacefully).

There is an immediacy to their workday and work concerns which stems, in great part, from the work of caring for surgical patients. 'Today's another day', a phrase which I heard several of the Sisters use, reveals that immediacy. Although their goals for individual patients and the ward transcend the time frame of a day, the Sisters make the ward work while they are on the ward, one day at a time. In this vein, the following discussion is largely organized around the flow of a day.

Allocating the work of the ward: matching nurses and patients

To accomplish the work of caring for all patients so that each may be helped towards recovery, the Ward Sisters need to maximize the potential of their staff. They do this by creating complementary work groups, assigning nurses to patients in such a way that patients get the care they need, and cueing nurses to the individual needs of patients.

The nursing staff

The Ward Sister is given a complement of qualified staff which is augmented by learners[4]. Qualified staff include ward sisters, staff nurses and on some wards, enrolled nurses. At the time of the study, on most wards there was only one ward sister; on four of the study wards there were two. The staff were deployed by the Sister according to the anticipated work flow on the early and the late shifts[5]. On some wards the staff nurses rotated onto nights (an internal rotation). While on a several-week night rotation, the staff nurse was removed from the 'off duty'[6], or work-hour sheet. She reported, as do the other night staff, to the night sisters. Recently, the staffing of the night shift has become the responsibility of the ward sister, and she has 24-hour responsibility and accountability for the ward and its staffing. At the time of the study, however, the Sisters usually did not know who was coming onto the night shift. This separation of responsibility for staffing the ward on days and nights created particular issues of continuity in patient care which are discussed later.

In one of the hospitals at the time of the study, learner nurses made up a large proportion of the nursing workforce on the surgical wards. Learner nurses included students who were studying towards their registration in General Nursing, Mental Handicap Nursing or Mental Nursing (first level nurses) and pupils who were studying to become second level or enrolled nurses. The learner nurses in both study hospitals were from one of two colleges of nursing and midwifery and one university nursing programme. The colleges controlled the allocation of students to the wards, so their numbers fluctuated. As the wards depended upon them for staffing purposes, when the numbers were low, the ward was short staffed.

Most of the wards in this study were used for the initial surgical nursing experience in the students' first year (13 weeks) and for the senior management experience (8–9 weeks). Some of the wards were used for surgical specialty experience or for 'unallocated' periods (4–5 weeks). Three wards in the study (orthopaedics and the two ear, nose and throat surgery wards) were sites for the post-basic course in their specialty and often had a post-basic student on the ward for several weeks at a time.

Part-time housekeepers or ward clerks performed clerical functions such as ordering supplies and equipment, making up patients' charts, and doing some of the paper work which accompanies patient admission and discharge. As with almost all the positions in the ward, when the ward clerkess was on maternity, illness or annual leave (the equivalent of vacation and statutory holidays) she was not replaced and the workload fell to the Ward Sister. Nursing assistants and orderlies (on the male wards) completed the complement of untrained staff.

On many of the wards there was only one auxiliary worker. As an experienced, long-term worker, the auxiliary was often a valuable, know-ledgeable resource to the ward. A domestic worker on each ward assisted with preparing meals and ward cleaning, but reported to a housekeeping or cleansing department. The Ward Sister generally made sure that there was a good working relationship with this person as the nursing staff had to take on aspects of their workload when he or she was absent.

Aside from the Sister and the auxiliary workers (and on some wards, the enrolled nurses), the workforce at the time of the study was inexperienced and transient. Most qualified nurses remained on the ward for only a year or so before moving to other nursing fields such as district nursing, intensive care or midwifery. To have a staff nurse on the ward for more than 2 years was a rarity. For many years, nurses have been expected to move on to 'broaden their horizons' in courses or in other nursing fields. For learners and some staff nurses, work on a particular ward may be a necessary interlude in their plans to complete a course or gain sufficient experience to be able to work in a different specialty. They are 'just passing through' (Melia 1987). With changes in employment prospects for nurses, this ethos has only recently begun to change. At the time of the study, several of the wards had only very junior staff nurses; the Ward Sister was the only experienced nurse on the ward. Such a workforce has considerable impact on the work of the Ward Sister.

Creating complementary work groups

Anticipating the workload and the capacity of the available nurses, the Ward Sisters arrange the 'off duty'[6] to allow for 'adequate cover'. They take into consideration the strengths and weaknesses of the nurses who will be working together. For instance, Sr Grant assigns a group of nurses who may have difficulty getting through the work, and who may not be too observant of patient needs, on a day in which the workload is less demanding. She schedules herself to work the following shift, so she catches needs and problems which may have been left unaddressed (W7D5: 1). Often the Ward Sister assigns herself to work with the most inexperienced nurses so she can support them with her experience, and provide a level of safety not possible otherwise. In scheduling the nurses' off duty, the Ward Sisters attempt to maximize the potential of the staff to meet the needs of the patients.

Allocating the work

In allocating the work of the ward, the Sisters aim to make the best use of resources, meeting the patients' individual care needs and the nurses' needs for a challenging but not overwhelming work assignment. They strive for flexibility yet suitability. The Sisters consider patient assignment to be one of their most important jobs.

Sr Grant: I make up an allocation of staff to patients and that's one of the most important parts of the day because if you do that well, your morning will run smoothly, your students will learn; your patients will be well cared for. You do it badly then everything falls apart. (Int. 7-1: 9–10)

Although all of the Sisters make a form of patient assignment, the shape is unique to each ward. Patient length of stay, the physical layout of the ward and patient procedures figure into the

particular form. On vascular surgery wards, where few patients go to theatre each day and patients stay from a week to a year, nurses are assigned to specific patients on the early shifts. On other wards, where patient turnover is quicker and more patients are going to theatre, the location of patients is a greater factor in their assignment.

Often a more senior nurse and a junior nurse will be assigned a group of patients, for example, 'You've got rooms 1–6', or 'You take the right side'. As patients are placed in particular rooms or beds according to their nursing care needs and their stage of recovery, what sounds like a physical space assignment is actually an assignment of patients. This mode of assignment is also common on the late shift when there are fewer nurses.

Continuity for patients is provided in ways which suit the patients and their environment. In the gynaecology ward, a team of nurses is assigned to care for patients of each team of surgeons operating on particular days. The nurses continue to care for these patients for up to a week of their stay. On the ear, nose and throat wards, where between 10 and 20 patients go to theatre each day, the patient assignment is linked to the theatre list[7]. Two or three nurses are assigned to 'pre-op and post-op'. Although it could be construed as task allocation, two nurses prepare the patients for theatre, take them to theatre and care for them following their operation. Usually the nurses assigned to pre- and post-op are a staff or enrolled nurse and a learner, which allows for supported learning while accomplishing the work. There is continuity of care for the patients, and an efficiency of workflow that allows fewer nurses to manage a larger workload.

Frequently, the necessary number of nurses is not there or the workload increases unexpectedly. Flexibility becomes the byword. One Sister describes the assignments she makes in these situations as we 'all pitch in'. For example, on one weekday early shift the Sister, two first-year students and an auxiliary (in the morning) are responsible for the care of 20 patients, most of whom are on bedrest.

Sr Aitkin: So you just do what you have to do. I could have been criticized maybe for the WAY that I ran the ward last Friday. I used the Resident to take patients for their [invasive procedures], to a different department, and to go and collect them for me, because . . . I couldn't go. I couldn't leave the ward and a first year couldn't go. And so the doctor did it.

One of the sickest ladies I had in the ward at that time, I had the auxiliary look after because I knew that she would do it the way I wanted it done; that she would report to me anyway if there was any change [. . .] I knew the first year would be too frightened to look after this particular lady. And the lady didn't come to any harm. She was very well cared for and everything was fine.

But I could have been criticized for doing that. But to me that was the only way I could manage the ward that morning. We all had a super morning. Everybody worked very hard and it all went very well. But it wasn't right. [laugh] (Int. 1-2: 29)

In one of the study hospitals, the Sisters experience many shifts such as this one. They are able to manage in such situations by virtue of their experience: knowing the capacity and strengths of their staff, anticipating the workload and flow of work through the shift, and knowing how to maximize the efforts of all their staff. However, in these circumstances, junior nurses take on more responsibility, with less supervision. They cope 'beyond what they should be expected to do' (W2D1: 1).

Preparing nurses to care for individuals

It is usual practice on the study wards for a nurse to begin work on a ward and to take a fair share of the workload on his/her first shift. Hence, the Ward Sisters become adept at introducing a new student or permanent staff member to the ward in a very short period of time and amidst the regular ward demands. A stark example of this is when Sr Grant orientates a new, first-year student to the ward in a period of 5 minutes before the late shift starts and while a moribund patient is admitted to the ward from Accident and Emergency. She is shown the most salient things in the ward so she can begin to function quickly and safely. Her questions about making off duty requests, her learning objectives, who will support her and who will assess her performance are anticipated and addressed immediately (W7D2-1: 2–3). Sr Grant pairs her with a staff nurse for the next two shifts, giving them patients who offer opportunities to learn some basic care practices on the ward. The staff nurse will continue to serve

as a source of support and continuity for the learner throughout her placement on the ward.

However, perhaps the most important way in which the Ward Sisters prepare the nurses for the care of the patients and for managing their workload is through their guidance at the hand-over report and during patient assignment. At the change of shift, the nurse in charge of the previous shift tells the nurse in charge of the oncoming shift (and others who may be present) about the patients, organizational arrangements and incidents which have occurred on the shift. Handover reports are not only used to pass information on from one shift to another. They also provide an opportunity for nurses to explore some patient problems and decide how best to manage these, to catch up on organizational or policy changes, and to relate how particular patient or organizational problems were solved. At this time, the Sisters give the patient assignment, telling about each patient. They pass on expectations about standards of care and help the learners and junior staff nurses to extend their knowledge of patients. Handovers are a key time in which the organizational culture of nursing on the ward is articulated and transmitted (Lelean 1973, Parker et al 1992, O'Brien & Pearson 1993). The Sisters cue the staff about what kind of information is valuable and worth passing on, and what comprises surgical nursing practice.

When Sr Aitkin gives nurses their assignments they hear about the patient as a person. With occasional reference to the patient's kardex, she often gives a short history of the patient's condition at home and in the hospital, gives some relevant facts about the condition or operation, the current goals for the patient's care and some specific things which the nurse must watch for, or attend to.

Mrs Muir :: 83 :: had a phenol sympathectomy :: She has been with us for some time :: She has a pre-gangrenous right foot :: She is a widow :: She has a grand niece who shows warm concern for her :: :: She is mentally alert from the waist up :: Her main concern is her cat :: We are aiming to get her to be with her cat :: get her to Rehabilitation Hospital :: We've even discussed Part 4 Accommodation :: She's fairly happy :: It is interesting, when I sat down to talk to her about her rehabilitation, she asked for tissue but she didn't use it :: She had a phenol on her other leg 11 years ago, and she asked 'Why isn't it working this time?' I said, 'You're 11 years older'. :: She needs a lot of encouragement :: She's a great churchgoer :: I watched her neighbour yesterday, organizing her bedside :: :: :: She can have a bath if she wants to get out of bed :: Her toe is blackened :: It may drop off :: The phenol has helped :: She walks with a zimmer :: She veers to the left while she is walking with people :: She may have had a wee stroke :: She can sit out of bed :: (W1D2-2: 5)

By telling about the patient as an active person in a family with interests and concerns, Sr Aitkin conveys the view that patients are people whose time in hospital is an interlude in their normal life. She alerts the student to some of Mrs Muir's interests which could serve as the topic of conversation and a point upon which to establish a relationship. She also interprets the symptoms which Mrs Muir is experiencing and alerts the nurse to potential changes and their meaning. When time permits, Sr Aitkin may take up to an hour to give this type of report on each patient to all the nurses, but feels it is worthwhile because:

Sr Aitkin: [. . .] these people are in for so long, it's very important to try and make the report interesting and make them think about the cat. (Int. 1-3: 18)

Although other Sisters may not take the same amount of time on their reports, the flavour of their assignments is the same. With differing amount of detail, depending upon the experience of the nurses, the Sisters point out specific, salient aspects of care. The Sisters place the nurses' work in a context of the patient's overall recovery process and help the nurses to understand the reasons for their actions. During the handover and patient assignment, the Sisters not only allocate the workload, but also help the nurses to learn about the patients' conditions and operations and, most importantly, encourage them to think about their patients as people.

Planning the care: having a clear agenda

Organizing the workflow of the ward is dependent upon planning the nursing care for individual patients, which in turn is intertwined with the medical plans and practices. Planning for care of the patient is the focus of the medical rounds which happen at least once daily.

To contribute to those rounds and to plan for the workflow of patient care, the Ward Sister makes an assessment of each patient early in the shift. Although she receives information on each patient at the handover report, the Ward Sister needs to 'see' the patients for herself before making rounds with the doctors. In the early part of the shift and at the handover report, the Ward Sister gets an overview of the ward, a sense of what has been happening and how the staff on the previous shift have been managing.

The Sisters' initial patient round is usually combined with at least one other activity. One Ward Sister receives the handover report from the night shift nurse at the patient's bedside. She is able to ask specific questions, she can say, 'Good morning' to the patients, she can see how they look and can find out from them how they are feeling. Another gives out the breakfasts:

She gives different bowls for cereal, depending on how agile the person is likely to be with the spoon. She does not spend a lot of time with each patient and no more than a look at the patients who have come in overnight and are fasting [for theatre], but I get the feeling she is doing her first of the morning assessment. She [checks out their circulation and range of motion], she finds out who is brighter or sicker than the day before, she finds out who is hungry today but wasn't yesterday, she finds out how easy or hard some people are to rouse; she finds out if [a long-term depressed patient] is cheerful or not. (W3D4: 1)

Assessing patients at this time is not a unitary activity, nor purely one of observation. The Sisters interact with the patients, suggest activities for the day, and hear patients' questions and concerns about future plans. They see how the nurses are beginning to organize their own work. From this early round, the Sisters bring to the rounds with the doctors specific concerns about each patient, their overall impression of the patients and how the nurses are carrying out the plans of care.

The focus of the surgical rounds is the doctors' plan of care. The Sisters bring any concerns about symptoms, the effects of the current plan, and possibilities for discharge to the doctors for their attention, investigation or referral. As 'a seeker after information' (Int. 7-3: 22), the Sisters come with knowledge of the patients on the ward and the problems they are having which need to be addressed.

Most of the rounds which I observed were

characterized by joint planning between the Ward Sisters and their senior doctors. In most cases there is a shared view of the patients and the goals for care, but in some instances there are different understandings about the goal or the patients' potential. This most often happens when planning for discharge or when a patient does not respond to surgical treatment and is dying. It is usually the Sister who works to get them into synchrony again, working to get 'everyone round to a SHARED view' (Int. 7-3: 27). Gaining a 'shared view' is possible because of the Sisters' authority in the ward and the respect and collegiality which underlies the relationship between the senior doctors and the Ward Sisters.

As medical and nursing spheres of action sometimes overlap, the consultants and Ward Sisters have tacit understandings about boundaries of practice, based on mutual trust and respect. That respect allows the Ward Sisters to push those boundaries in situations where they may hold different views on the needs of a patient. In one situation, Sr Grant asks the Resident to refer a patient to rehabilitation while the consultant is on holiday because she knows the consultant is reluctant to let the patient leave the ward. Although she is 'very hesitant to put the wheels into motion without discussing it with him' (Int. 7-3: 3), she does.

Sr Grant: I didn't want to get into the situation of us having his wounds healed, then deciding we'd apply for rehab. And then having to wait a month, kicking his heels really until the bed was ready. (Int. 7-3: 3)

When the consultant returns from holiday, he makes a point of saying he has noticed the referral. Sr Grant tells him 'I took the liberty of arranging for [rehabilitation]' (W7D2-1: 12) and tells him her reasoning. Sr Grant describes it thus, 'I think it was an acknowledgement by us both that I was just pushing the boundary a little' (Int. 7-3: 4). Working together in everyday practice, the Ward Sisters and their medical staff find, test and reaffirm or change the boundaries of practice.

Following medical rounds, the Sisters call the nurses together to receive any new information from them and to give them an update on their patients. Although some of the work generated from the decisions made in rounds is undertaken by the doctors, much falls to the nurses.

Getting on with the work: keeping one jump ahead

To get on with the work of a shift, the Ward Sisters organize the flow of patients into and out of the ward, and help the nurses to organize their own workloads. They keep the workflow moving by monitoring nursing practices and the care the patients receive, providing intervention, support and back-up where needed. To accomplish these things, the Ward Sisters literally have to keep 'one jump ahead'.

Sr Calder: [...] I know I have always got to be a jump ahead. To maintain this workload, and get as much as possible out ... of the little we've got. (Int. 3-3: 17)

Organizing the patients and the nurses

On some of the wards, 12 or more people are discharged and as many again are admitted into the ward in a morning. To achieve a smooth patient turnover, the discharged patients have to be ready to leave early. Sr Calder has a reputation in the hospital for being extraordinarily skilled in managing the high turnover of her ward. She anticipates which patients are likely to be going home and includes that in her assignment to the nurses. For example:

Mr Tennant :: sliced the top of the left index finger off :: If it's a usual finger, three doses of IV antibiotics and home :: No reason he can't get up. He has marked staining on the bandage so he'll have his bandage covered today. (W3D5: 3)

Before the doctors appear for rounds, Sr Calder makes follow-up appointments for those patients who she is sure will be discharged, but delays making appointments for those about whom she is less sure. She also has the discharge letters prepared for the Resident, save for any unique discharge instructions and prescriptions. After rounds:

[...] Sr Calder then sets about to discharge those patients whom [the Registrar] has said could go home. [The Resident] signs the letters [which also serve as the requisitions to Pharmacy for medications for home] and the housekeeper takes them down to Pharmacy. The drugs come up amazingly quickly. Sr Calder gives those patients that don't require antibiotics pain killers from the medication trolley [a bubble pack of Distalgesic™]. Sr Calder tells me, 'The minute they are discharged these young ones want to

go. I need the tablets under control by that time'.
(W3D3: 6)

Knowing the patients, the doctors and their practices and how the hospital support departments work, enables Sr Calder to keep one jump ahead. She knows that once many of the young patients have received word from the doctors, they will not wait long for their discharge letter, follow-up appointment and medications (which are usually antibiotics and analgesics). She also knows that the Pharmacy Department workload is heavy in the middle of the morning so she ensures that the discharge prescriptions from her ward are among the first filled.

Through Sr Calder's anticipation and quick action, by mid-morning the ward is ready for more new patients. Her pacing and timing is suited to the patients and situation of the ward. On other wards, where the pace of turnover is not so high, and where patients are not so apt to leave without the necessary medications, this fast pace is not essential. However, on all wards, the Sisters plan ahead for unexpected admissions. They follow a maxim of being prepared: 'You must always have a bed in a prime situation in the ward, [. . .] ready [. . .] if you can' (Int. 2-3: 21). Being ready includes thinking ahead to the patients who may be coming in.

Sr Aitkin: 'So that they have the jugs and glasses on the locker and the chairs by the bed. [. . .] It looks as if you're expecting them. I don't like the patient to come in and think, 'Now where am I going to go?' (Int. 1-3: 27–28)

Coming with an understanding of the patients and the workflow which is broader and deeper than that of inexperienced nurses, the Ward Sisters see different priorities and act accordingly.

Sr Grant: [. . .] I start to [. . .] strip a bed and make up a bed for the expected admission. Whereas the student nurse. That patient hasn't arrived yet. That patient's nothing to worry about yet. It hasn't happened. She has other priorities. She's not [. . .] looking ahead in the same way that I am. So she finds it difficult to understand why Sister wants to stop and strip and make up this fresh bed when she's got things that she feels that she needs to do first. [. . .]
And it happens [. . .] the other way around. The student nurse who's not sure if she's heard her blood pressure correctly, who would like to have it checked by me, when I know this is a routine observation and

the patient is WELL. And I'm not too concerned. It's a low priority for me to check that blood pressure when I've got so many other pressing things to do. But that blood pressure's very important to that student nurse. (Int. 7-1: 12–13)

When experienced staff nurses are not available, a good part of the Ward Sisters' time is spent helping the nurses to become organized and to set and reset priorities in a way that accomplishes the work, while providing a quality of care to the patient. Unable to rely upon taken-for-granted understandings, the Sisters often need to make their priorities and actions explicit. This can feel like 'pushing' and 'driving' the students and junior staff (W9D3: 1).

Keeping the workflow going with the patient at the centre

With a clear overview of the work to be done and the potential of each patient, the Sisters are able to combine actions, anticipate problems and coordinate activities, helping the nurses to achieve the goals of care for individual patients while addressing the needs of all. The Sisters learn how to 'use every minute you have, and not to waste one second of a nurse's time' (W9D3: 1). This does not come easily, particularly when there is an ever increasing workload and too few people to help.

The Sisters talk about 'cutting corners' in such situations. 'Cutting corners' is not easily defined, but central to its meaning is being flexible and paring down actions. The Ward Sisters are selective about which corners they cut and how they do it. They do not cut corners to save time in the short run, when the long-term effect is compromised recovery for a patient. On a very short staffed day, Sr Calder gets an elderly patient with a fractured humerus and infected chest up to sit in a chair before breakfast, so the arm benefits from postural traction and the patient breathes better (W3D2-2: 3). The Ward Sisters not only see the immediate task to be done, they have a broader plan for the patient and do what is necessary now to prevent complications later. They recognize what will and will not be time saving, taking this broader goal into their definition of what may be minimum nursing care. Sr Calder describes how she sees the work organization differently from her staff nurses.

Sr Calder: But they're not seeing it the same way as I see it. [. . .] Whereas they would see it — give him his breakfast in bed and then we'll be getting him up out of bed later. [to do his bath] [. . .] They would do breakfast first. They wouldn't see another job to do. (Int. 3-3: 27)

The Sisters understand their present actions as a part of a larger whole. They know where the patient is in the course of recovery, know where he has to get to and know what actions are required to get him there. It enables them to 'see another job to do'.

In times of staff shortage, sometimes only the highest priorities of care are accomplished.

Sr Grant: You constantly have to sort through priorities and decide what you can do now, what you can do later and what you won't be able to do. But there ARE things that you feel you should be doing. [. . .] It means that some important things like supervision of the nurse learners just goes by the board. It's more important that the patient is washed and moved and comfortable than it is for the student to be supervised. You just hope for the best. (Int. 7-1: 11–12)

The Sisters say they can manage by cutting corners for short periods of time, but on a longer term basis, this interferes with student supervision and thus the standards of care can suffer. Consequently, morale suffers too.

One of the several techniques used by the Ward Sisters to keep the workflow going for patient care is to maximize the effect of their experience. Sometimes it means that the nurses become something of an extension of the Sisters. When the man with postoperative bleeding needs diligent watching, Sr Jarvis is specifically directive. She cannot count on the student's independent judgement and action.

Sr Jarvis: And I felt it was up to me, not exactly to be looking after the patient on my own, but not relying on the nurse who WAS looking after the patient to pick up on the subtle changes that I was looking for. (Int. 10-2: 24)

The Sisters try to strike a balance between allowing the junior nurses independent action, and recognizing the needs of the patients and the nurses' limitations. As they give a report, help a student to become organized at a patient's

bedside, or do a procedure, the Sisters often say, 'The most important thing to remember is . . .' (W8D2-1: 8). In this way, the Sisters help the students attend to the most important concerns — the concerns to which they would be attending if they could be there.

When she does not have sufficient nursing staff who can act independently, the Ward Sister can be in a difficult position. All are affected as the Ward Sister attends to 'the one who needs me more than anybody else' (Int. 1-2: 19). On days such as these,

Sr Baxter: I can't observe as a manager that the patients are getting the proper care and that everything's flowing, that they've had their X-rays and that their IVs are going and that they are pain free. And these things can all be dealt with. If I can't observe that and there are no nurses to do it, then it doesn't happen. And then what you end up with is a patient who is uncomfortable or in pain. (Int. 2-1: 24)

At these times, it is far more difficult to retain an overview, to monitor and to intervene when necessary.

Surgical patients frequently require small procedures. The Ward Sisters try to make sure that the procedures are accomplished in a timely fashion and in a way that supports the patients' recovery. For instance, they are particular about when a person's urinary catheter is removed.

'Ask the night nurse to do an MSU so we can take the catheter out first thing in the morning. We do it that way rather than taking it out in the day so that if they piddle it is not at night which worries them. They will get it out of the way during the day.' (W1D1: 9)

They recognize that the incontinence which is likely to follow catheter removal is worrying to patients. A secondary consideration, but one which affects the care of others, is that during the day patients can more readily get to a toilet and there may not be the same requirement to change soiled beds.

Sometimes, the Sisters 'plant seeds' with patients, so they are ready for procedures or baths when the staff are ready. The Sisters consider that allowing patients to prepare for procedures and negotiating with them about when activities are done is not only respectful — it engenders cooperation. It also helps to keep the work flowing. 'You get more by going at their pace' (Int. 2-3: 6).

Ward Sisters coordinate procedures with the times that doctors are available to the patients. In the middle of a round, Sr Jarvis asks a staff nurse to 'do a residual on Mrs Lester so it is done before the doctors go, and maybe she can go home' (W10D1: 5). Coordinating action in this way allows the patient to be evaluated more quickly and keeps Mrs Lester from having to wait longer in hospital for the doctor to return to evaluate and discharge her. It also provides the potential for a bed to be available earlier than might otherwise be the case.

The Sisters also keep the work flowing by keeping one jump ahead of the doctors. Sr Hanna picks up on the results of the BCG (pregnancy) and ultrasound tests and begins to fast a woman who is most likely having a miscarriage and will need a dilatation and curettage. Her knowledge of the patient's history, the significance of the lab tests and likely medical practice means she can anticipate the required action. By beginning the preparations for theatre and by fasting the woman, she can get to theatre earlier. Potentially, this means less blood loss for the patient and, through speedier treatment, possibly an earlier return home.

In summary, the Sisters keep the work flowing through their own actions and by actively supporting the actions of others. They organize and coordinate the work and intervene where and when necessary to move things along. They continually revise priorities for care, keeping a finely tuned tension between the needs of individual patients and the needs of all.

Solving immediate problems with a view to the future

With a largely transient and inexperienced work-force, the Ward Sisters continually help junior medical and nursing staff solve immediate problems in a way that may help them to solve similar problems on their own in the future. The Sisters do not take on others' problems: they set the scene for doctors and nurses to take responsibility with support.

The Sisters routinely help junior nurses to interpret signs, symptoms and patient conditions.

At report [Nurse Melrose] hears that Mr Peters is to be 'on half hourlies until he is awake, or if you are concerned, on half hourlies for 2–3 hours'. About 3 hours later, Nurse Melrose asks Sr Jarvis a question about continuing Mr Peters on half hourly BP. Sr Jarvis is about to answer, when she says, 'What do you think?' Nurse Melrose says, 'I could stop,' and points to the BP going down into the 120/70 range. 'It is what he had pre-op.' Sr Jarvis says, 'Really?' (turning the sheet over and showing her the BP was higher) Sr Jarvis points to where it is higher, 'This could have been his pre-med and this because he was nervous'. Sr Jarvis turns the sheet back, pointing that the blood pressure trend is downward. She says, 'This is reason for carrying on. Take it once more and see how it stabilizes'. (W10D2: 11–12)

Guiding the student's observations and interpreting the patient's responses pre- and postoperatively, Sr Jarvis assists the nurse to consider the larger pattern and context of the patient's physiological response. Such interchanges were frequently observed with all of the Sisters.

The Sisters help the nurses learn to address problems directly.

[Sr Hanna is sitting in the ward doing] her charting :: Nurse Cotter comes up and asks her, 'What is this?', showing her a notation on the fluid balance sheet for [poorly written KCl] :: Sr Hanna: 'I don't know. I haven't a clue.' Nurse Cotter turns and goes off to the doctors' room. Bill [the Resident] comes back with her to Sr Hanna and says, 'It's KCl'. Sr Hanna: 'I know, but I'm not here all the time'. :: (W8D2-1: 19)

The Sisters set up situations for students to take responsibility in little things because they recognize the effect on the nurses' confidence and subsequent ability. Given the staffing situation on most of the study wards, even newly qualified staff nurses have to take charge of shifts. 'They don't have any choice' (W10D3: 12). The Sisters take various approaches to organizing the workload so that nurses gradually learn to take on more responsibility and are not overwhelmed and unable to function. On one ward that means giving a staff nurse or senior student responsibility for a team while the Sister retains overall responsibility for the ward. It 'allows her to learn how to do a sensible patient assignment' (Int. 10-3: 14). As the staff nurse is given responsibility for planning all the care for the group of patients, she has to begin to think differently about the extent of that care. Instead of thinking:

Sr Jarvis: 'We haven't got to worry about: Mr X needs a bath today and then he's got a such and such dressing to be done. That's him [. . .] done.' (Int. 10-3: 15)
The nurse has to realize that there is more to the patient's care:
Sr Jarvis: He might have a wife that's not well. The doctors might be thinking that he's ready to go home later in the week. What are we going to do about getting him home. Does he need an ambulance and this sort of thing. They suddenly have to consider that it wasn't just Mr X's personal hygiene and his wound healing that they have to deal with. It's all the other sides to him as well. (Int. 10-3: 15)

Taking responsibility for the care of a group of patients, the new staff nurse broadens her understanding of care and learns how to work with students.

The Sisters often give support and direction to junior medical staff. Decisions about admission and discharge are sometimes difficult for doctors to make. In the following situation Sr Grant discusses what she was thinking when she suggested an alternative admission arrangement to a new Registrar.

Sr Grant: Several things. One [. . .] I knew that we were basically discussing bed state. But the niceties of it washed over me. Secondly because he's new to the unit, he is perhaps more willing to accept patients that would be more appropriately admitted elsewhere. So that rang a bell immediately. Here we have a diabetic in a medical outpatient clinic. Usually these patients are admitted to medical wards, worked up and then brought over here if they require vascular surgery. So I thought [. . .] 'This really shouldn't come our way at all.' Thirdly that he wanted me to make a decision about when this patient would be admitted. Now that's not a nursing responsibility. And fourthly was the desire to help him out, because he was struggling. And it would have been easy to say, 'Well I have a bed today. Yes that's fine. Go ahead'.
M.M.:   Mm hmm. But you didn't do that.
Sr Grant: No, because the next time the same problem would crop up. And I might not necessarily have the bed. And he would not have discovered what the correct process was that way. (Int. 7-3: 9–10)

Sr Grant shows that she understands the situation new registrars often find themselves in regarding admitting non-straightforward patients. She gets under the surface of the request, acknowledging what he is asking, but recognizing that it would be an inappropriate admission. Had the patient been admitted to the ward, the Registrar's judgement would have been ques-

tioned by the senior medical staff. Sr Grant's knowledge of the usual admission practices allows her to help him solve a medical organizational problem and see that the patient gets an appropriate medical referral. The Registrar retains responsibility for the problem and learns to solve it.

Monitoring the quality of care and being a safety net

Where many of the nurses are inexperienced, and where frequently overworked junior doctors provide on-the-spot medical cover, the Ward Sisters play a vital role in monitoring and ensuring the quality of care, intervening when necessary. They provide a web of practices so that patients do not 'fall through the cracks' and are a safety net for the junior medical and nursing staff.

The Sisters watch the doctors and nurses as they go about their work, listen to them as they work together and with patients, ask questions about their knowledge and expectations for their care, and notice the effect of their actions on the patients. They pick up on errors, spot omissions, intervene when junior staff members are 'running into trouble' and seek assistance from more senior medical staff for decisions which are beyond the ability of the resident or registrar in the ward. Such monitoring and intervention is done with finesse, and in a manner which usually encourages ongoing communication and cooperation.

Making an accurate assessment of a patient's condition or activity tolerance is often difficult for inexperienced nurses.

While Sr Hanna is sitting at the desk in the ward writing her care plans, she is listening :: [. . .] to the [2 first year] nurses getting Mrs Han [a 33-year-old who went to theatre about 4 hours earlier for a laparoscopy] up to the commode. Sr Hanna asks, 'You weren't thinking of getting her up to the commode were you?' They say, 'Yes'. Sr Hanna: 'I think it is still early. Stay with her'. (W8D3: 17)

Sr Hanna acknowledges the students' assessment, gives her opinion and cautions them to stay with the patient to make their action safe. She questions their judgement and intervenes in a way which does not undermine their decision. In other situations, the Ward Sister may change the intervention. Sr Grant responds to a nurse's request for pain medication for a patient; when she takes the medication to him, she identifies that the pain is angina, not simply limb pain. Through her different assessment and subsequent intervention, Sr Grant ensures that appropriate, safe care is given. And, to help the nurse learn from her error, she discusses it with her afterwards (W7D2-2: 16).

The Ward Sisters also provide support for junior doctors. This happens during the lead-up to Mr Peet's surgery (see p 64). After Sr Ellis talks with Mr Peet and his family, the Resident, Dr Campbell, takes Mr Peet's cousin and her husband into his office to explain the planned surgery. After about 20 minutes, Sr Ellis goes to her office to get something to file and then to the doctor's office where Dr Campbell is talking to the couple.

She knocks [goes in] and puts the paper into the file. The conversation stops and Sr Ellis turns to join in it. They talk about the cousin's daughter being called and coming in to see him this evening. The couple thank the doctor and go back to Mr Peet.
Sr Ellis asks Dr Campbell how it went after they leave. He looks troubled and says :: 'They're saying the right words. The things are going round and round but you don't know if they're dropping into the right slots.' Sr Ellis nods. As we go out of the room, she says to me, 'He's nice :: And he's only 24 :: it's hard for them'. (W5D2-1: 15)

While she recognizes that the family needs to hear about the plans for Mr Peet from a doctor, Sr Ellis is aware of Dr Campbell's inexperience and his need for support.

Sr Ellis: I went in just to look and go out again if I thought ... But I felt he'd got too deep. [...] And I could sense that going in. [...] So that's why we went in, to try and wind it up. Because I thought, 'Well you can make things worse by going on and on into minute details and that'. You know, there's only so much that people can take in.
And I could see just from his face and brow. [chuckle] The way the conversation was sort of dry and ... I knew he'd sort of done the nitty gritty part of the chat. So I'm really protecting him, more than anything else. (Int. 5-3: 24)

As well as tangible support for the junior doctor, Sr Ellis' action could also be considered supportive for the family as she prevents the situation from deteriorating.

The Sisters set up mechanisms for minimizing omissions, for ensuring that things 'don't fall through the cracks'. They recognize the difficulties the nurses may have in attending to the myriad of details involved in caring for acute care surgical patients. One such mechanism is a wound check book in which all the patients whose wounds need checking are listed.

Sr Inglis [...] says it might be old fashioned, but she found that nurses were missing it, and the junior students' assessments couldn't be trusted. 'For example, see, Mr Breen's was red, not "fine" like [first year student] charted. I like the senior nurse or the nurse-in-charge to go round to see all the wounds ... Perhaps it should be picked up in the nursing process but .... Wounds are important, they can go wrong.' (W9D1: 11)

Although such a list could be seen as an indicator of a routine task approach, here it serves to ensure a quality of care to individuals where many of the caregivers are inexperienced. The Sisters help junior nurses learn to build in regular assessments of their patients by linking this with other aspects of their care. To help maintain a patient's fluid intake, Sr Inglis advises the students to ask their patients to take a drink each time they use the commode (W9D2: 3). Sometimes Sisters keep patients on formal monitoring longer than necessary, as a technique to ensure that the nurses regularly observe the patients. The ENT Sisters keep some newly post-op patients on half-hourly recordings slightly longer than needed so the nurses regularly go into the rooms to observe them. With the number of patients on the ward, the inexperience of many staff and their knowledge of human fallibility, the Ward Sisters ensure that the risks to patients are minimized.

Ensuring continuity of nursing care

The Ward Sisters seek to achieve a consistent standard of care for each patient throughout all shifts. As discussed earlier, they accomplish this in part through staff allocation and patient assignment. However, ensuring continuity of care through the night shift presents the greatest challenge (Williams 1989). At the time of the study, for 11 hours each day, the Ward Sister did not hold formal authority or responsibility for the care of the patients, but remained accountable for their overall care. On many wards, an internal rotation of a staff nurse to the night shift promoted continuity of care, but it was only one nurse at a time and did not address other issues of formal authority. Continuity of care was also difficult to maintain with the constant turnover of students and junior medical staff. The Ward Sisters sometimes found themselves orientating new staff to the ward on a weekly basis. While ward manuals and guidelines for such things as patient admissions helped to provide a continuous thread, it was the Ward Sisters' expectations and everyday practices which enabled continuity and maintenance of a particular standard of care.

The handover reports at the change of shift provide glimpses of such practices. In preparation for a change of shift, the Ward Sister identifies who is coming on, the strengths they may have and/or the potential difficulties they may encounter. For example, when patients require diligent watching and the ward is busy, the Ward Sister may check to see if those coming on to the night shift have the capacity to cope or whether extra staff should be requested.

Sr Jarvis: This gentleman wasn't well and I thought that he needed a close eye kept on him. [. . .] And it mattered to me who was going to be coming on because this was getting near to the time I was going to be handing over. And I had to think about whether they were going to cope. Or whether they were going to need somebody else. And in actual fact the next gentleman that came back on the same day, also had problems with bleeding. So we had quite a lot to think about.
  So that was something else I considered, was the staffing and whether or not they were going to manage.
M.M.:   And what did you conclude?
Sr Jarvis: And in actual fact, I concluded that they would be all right. As the staff nurse who was coming on was quite capable. And she's always good to students, if you like, and the mix was . . .
M.M.:   The mix was good. Mm hmm.
Sr Jarvis: Mm hmm. (Int. 10-2: 29–30)

It is not only the numbers which concern the Sisters, but the quality and mix of the staff; their capacity to deal successfully with the particular patients on the ward. This concern reflects the Ward Sisters' recognition of the fact that the quality of nursing care is directly related to the nurses giving that care.

To help prepare the oncoming nurses, the Sisters often cue them at the handover report about what to expect. Reports to unknown or inexperienced staff are often very detailed. The Ward Sisters give specific directions about what to look for with particular patients and reasons for unusual or common but necessary procedures, for example, 'He's having frequent oral care because he's fasting' (W9D3: 21). They give oncoming nurses specific directions.

Sr Jarvis: I said to her that I wasn't happy with his wound at all. And I thought that it hadn't healed and it was gradually coming apart. And to make sure that she let the Registrar see it when he came back on the ward round that evening. Explained that we'd taken out one of the deep tension sutures, and emphasized to her that we really had to make sure that they kept a close eye on it. And to re-change the dressing again on the evening shift. (Int. 10-2: 13)

The Ward Sisters organize themselves and their senior staff to give the most continuity and support to inexperienced nurses. They alter the workload where they can to ease the burden on inexperienced staff; and sometimes alert medical and senior nursing staff to the inexperience of the staff telling them to expect calls and to be supportive. In sum, they attempt to ensure a continuity and a quality of care to patients which transcends the shifts that they themselves are on.

Creating a caring ward

Creating and maintaining smoothly functioning, caring wards within the complex and ever-changing organization of a teaching hospital is an ongoing challenge for the Ward Sisters. Primarily, they work to create an atmosphere on the ward which is healing for the patients and supportive for the nurses. This is accomplished in part by building their largely transient and junior workforce into a working team and by putting professional and educational supports into place which assist the nurses to develop their practice. Wards cannot work without necessary services, equipment and supplies. To obtain these in a system which does not always work smoothly, the Ward Sisters have developed ways of working with other hospital services and departments. This points to perhaps one of the more difficult aspects of the Ward Sisters' practice, reconciling overall organizational change and planning with the needs and concerns of the staff and patients on the ward. As leaders and managers of the ward, the Ward Sisters are pivotal in determining links to the wider organization.

The Ward Sisters play a central part in creating the ward atmosphere, the feeling of the ward.

Sr Hanna: [...] I would like to think that every person that comes in the door of the ward is aware of that atmosphere and I would like to think that that atmosphere is there because of the way that I run the ward; the relationships that I form with the medical staff and the relationships I form with my permanent nursing staff. (Int. 8-1: 1)

In a ward, the atmosphere enables or constrains people's actions. When the ward atmosphere is a good one, both the patients and the nurses benefit (McGhee 1961, Orton 1981). On Sr Aitkin's ward, a patient who had been on a number of wards told me, 'You can tell a happy place . . . It is happy from the top. This is a happy ward' (W1D1: 5). Students also commented to me that the study wards were 'good' wards to be on. It seems that the little things which Sisters did or set up to happen were significant in creating the atmosphere.

The comportment of the Ward Sisters influences the atmosphere. A patient described Sr Aitkin: 'She exudes confidence . . . She has confidence in us' (W1D1: 5). The Sisters share of themselves, and allow for openness and caring amongst others in the ward. Their work pattern and style help to create a ward atmosphere and influence other nursing staff.

Sr Grant: [...] I think they tend to follow your pattern. Particularly if they're new to their role. They will absorb everything you do. And your style to a certain extent. (Int. 7-3: 19–20)

It is mainly through their pattern and style of practices that the Ward Sisters build a largely transient and junior workforce into a working team. This is particularly so on the study wards of Hospital B where the Sister is often the only qualified staff nurse on any particular shift. At Hospital A, a solid core of permanent staff and proportionately fewer students give rise to slightly different practices. However, it is through everyday practices that the Sisters encourage students and junior staff nurses to join with the more experienced staff to become a working team.

All of the Sisters make a point of warmly welcoming new students, staff and nurses who are assigned to the ward for a single shift. Sr Aitkin talks about the patients and staff on the ward being all part of the 'family' of the ward 'while you are here'. Even I was introduced as 'part of the family for the week' (W1D1: 2). Although the students are considered to be 'just passing through' the ward, the Sisters provide personal support to many of them when their work on the ward provokes personal difficulties. Often older and more experienced than other nurses who have higher status, the auxiliaries and/or enrolled nurses sometimes need particular support.

Sr Hanna: And the whole atmosphere in the ward can be influenced by a strong personality that's not in a good mood if you want to put it. And so it's important that if you see this happening you try and do something about it quite quickly. And 'cause I always think it's infectious when one person starts getting grumpy it can easily be passed on to the next person. So you've got to make sure that it doesn't escalate. (Int. 8-1: 16)

Recognizing the early signs of a bad mood or being troubled, the Ward Sisters intervene to give the person some support. It may be to 'say something to them that will make them feel better'. Or it may be to take the grumbles 'off her', to make sure she gets to coffee early, or to offer the opportunity to talk over a quiet cup of coffee. Through these and other forms of tangible supports, the Ward Sisters care for their staff and students and bring about a functioning team of nurses.

Professional and educational supports often take the form of reference material such as standard care plans, information sheets, books and articles. The Sisters make use of the talents of clinical teachers, senior staff nurses and nurses on induction or professional development courses. On some wards, the Sisters arrange for the staff nurses to give regular tutorials to the students. They negotiate post-basic, induction and professional development course projects which are of benefit to the ward as well as to the nurse. On one ward, the Sister capitalized on a staff nurse's interest in patient education and encouraged her to write information sheets for the patients about common procedures and tests. The Sister smoothed the path with the surgeons, and the staff nurse was able to learn and grow while providing something of importance to the patients.

Despite the busyness of the wards, the Sisters arrange for students to go to theatre to see surgical procedures. 'It gives them an idea of what the patients go through and why they have pain' (W3D4: 3). Students and staff nurses are also given opportunities to become involved with the activities of patient self-help groups.

Even though these supports for learning and practice are sometimes unevenly implemented, they are a means through which the nurses' skills can be enhanced and professional contributions fostered.

To carry out the work of the ward, sufficient supplies and services are required and it is not always easy to obtain these. Services include, for example, having a bed pan cleanser repaired or replaced or having specially-ordered patients' meals delivered.

Sr Hanna: You know you cannot depend on just doing something and it will happen or requesting something to happen. It is never easy. It's always complicated. (Int. 8-1: 19)

To help the process of getting supplies, the Ward Sisters get to know the people in other departments and how they can be best approached. Where the normal systems break down or an unusual request needs to be made, the Sisters use these relationships to obtain the services required for patients. The importance of having adequate supplies on the ward is not underestimated by the Ward Sisters. They also get to know the usual flow of supplies from other departments. One Sister makes a point of hoarding linen several days before holiday weekends when linen supplies are unreliable and generally low. As the system of linen delivery changes, so does her hoarding. She maintains a flexible stance but protects the needs of her ward first.

The Ward Sisters work to keep the disruption and uncertainty of the organizational environment away from the ward. The study coincided with the introduction of Unit Management in the Health Board and corresponding organizational changes in the hospitals. Prior to and during the 10 months of field work, the Sisters coped with organizational uncertainty, changes in reporting structure, changes in the provision of services by departments such as laundry, domestics (cleansing) and portering. One ward moved location and combined with another ward, another changed the type of patients and a third was the subject of plans to change to a 5-day ward. In addition, there was a period of labour unrest, with several work stoppages by health care unions protesting against insufficient health funding.

Sr Hanna: All right it may go on all around about you, but I don't want that infiltrating into the ward. I like to try to keep the atmosphere different in the ward. (Int. 8-1: 19)

The atmosphere which is sought for the ward is one of caring and concern. The Sisters seek to protect the ward against the 'stresses and strains' of the organization. Although they have a great deal of clinical authority inside their wards, most of the Sisters say they are often not consulted, nor involved in early stages of decision-making regarding nursing policy and organizational changes.

During such times, the Ward Sisters feel powerless and frustrated, as they are expected to make changes work even when they think the changes may be wrong-headed. At times they 'Ignore half of them, I think' (Grp. Int. 1: 37). At other times they express their concerns to the nursing officer, or only accept limited responsibility. In accepting and making changes, they operate from the perspective of what is best for the patient and the staff, followed by doing what is necessary to survive in the organization. Being a semi-permeable membrane — by using their clinical authority in the ward, and cushioning the impact of organizational stresses — the Ward Sisters help nurses get on with their job of helping patients towards recovery.

THE NATURE OF PRACTICE

This chapter provides the context of the Sisters' practice from which we can examine the process of practising nursing and of becoming experienced. The argument thus far has been that experience is not static, but is fluid, multifaceted and inextricably linked to ongoing, moment-by-moment everyday practice. In this chapter I have argued that the Sisters' practice is patient-centred and complex, geared towards multi-layered goals.

The Sisters' practice and experience are influenced by the complex, ever-changing nature of their surgical wards. Centring their care firmly on the patient, the patient's stay is the frame for the Sisters' practices with individuals and their families. These practices, however, are always within the context of making the ward work for all of the patients. While their care of individual patients is geared to each patient's unique course of hospitalization and recovery, the Sisters approach the work of the ward on a day-by-day basis. Although the temporal frameworks for the care of individuals and the work of the ward differ, the Sisters always practise with an eye to the future and an understanding of the past.

The Sisters' practice does not seem to have separate clinical, management and teaching components as much of the literature would suggest (cf. Pembrey 1980, Orton 1981, Fretwell 1982). When their practices are closely examined separate components are not evident at all, not even components with 'close interrelationships' among them (Runciman 1983). Rather, the Sisters' practice is complex and multifaceted. They often accomplish many goals simultaneously.

The Sisters are sensitive to the patients' needs from the beginning of the patients' stay in hospital. The Sisters present themselves and create the possibility for a trusting relationship with the Sisters and the other nurses. Such a relationship is critical if the patients' stay in hospital is to be 'a smooth passage'. The Sisters do not stand apart from the patients. Rather, they engage the patient in a personal, yet professional relationship. This is the point at which the Sisters begin to get to know the patients within the context of their hospitalization and surgery (MacLeod 1993). Knowing the patients, and their particular responses to surgery and hospitalization, enables the Sisters to tailor their practices to the individual. However, the Sisters give only a small amount of the direct care on a ward themselves.

Nursing care on a ward is a group endeavour. When patient problems are complex and require expert intervention, the Sisters will provide care themselves. For the most part, however, they use their expertise to plan, monitor and evaluate the care that others give. Their efforts are geared toward assisting their largely inexperienced and junior workforce to provide good quality care to individuals. The Sisters accomplish this through their practices in allocating the work, preparing the nurses to care for patients and supporting the nurses in giving that care. Sometimes directive, their practices are primarily facilitative. The Sisters actively work to create an atmosphere in the ward which is supportive for both the patients and the nurses (and doctors) caring for them. They guide the nurses in learning to recognize salient aspects of a situation and to take appropriate action. Characteristically, the Sisters work with junior nurses (and doctors) in such a way that they are supported while taking responsibility and learning to solve problems.

The Sisters continually strive to provide the best quality of care for patients that they are able to under the circumstances in which they find themselves. To this end, they keep in mind the broad picture of the work of the ward and the course of recovery for the patient. They sometimes have to 'cut corners' but find ways to do it that minimize the negative effects on patients. The Sisters act as safety nets for patients and for junior and inexperienced staff: monitoring practice, preventing and picking up on the errors and omissions which inevitably occur. They develop a web of practices which helps to prevent patients from 'falling through the net' and missing out on necessary care.

The Sisters' practices are directed towards ensuring continuity for individual patients while ensuring care for all. They strive to keep the patients' families in synchrony with the changes in the patients' condition; they work to keep the doctors and nurses in synchrony about the plans for patient progress. Ensuring consistency in the care of patients from shift to shift with a continually changing workforce is accomplished, sometimes with considerable difficulty, through clear communication at handover reports, as well as through clear expectations about the standard of care communicated through their everyday practices.

As the linchpin between the ward and the broader organization, the Sisters develop relationships with support departments and services which smooth the process of obtaining the supplies, equipment and services that the ward and the patients require. They are not always successful in these endeavours, and are sometimes not as involved in organizational planning as they would like to be. Nevertheless, the Sisters attempt to keep the stresses and strains of the organization from negatively influencing the caring atmosphere of the ward.

The discussion in this chapter reveals the importance of the context in determining the meanings of everyday practices. The meanings of the Sisters' practices derive from the ongoing situation of which they are a part. Thus the understanding we have of surgical nursing from the nursing textbooks (e.g. Alexander et al 1994), and of ward sister practice from the research literature (e.g. Pembrey 1980) are but shadows of what actually goes on. The patient and the on-going situation, the two essential elements of nursing practice, are overlooked in these accounts.

If we accept that nursing practice is contextual and relational then it seems important to examine more closely how the Sisters go about the process of practising surgical nursing.

Notes

[1] Although the primary goal is to help patients towards recovery, not all patients recover. Helping patients to die peacefully is an important part of the Sisters' practice. It is under-represented in this discussion as I have opted to focus on recovery.

[2] The medication orders and sheets are kept on a clipboard at the base of the patients' beds and are accessible to them.

[3] The term 'beds' is used here because with admissions, discharges, day surgery patients, and emergency and outpatients, there may be more patients than beds at any one time.

[4] For example, on a 21 bed general surgery ward, the staff complement at the time of the study was 1 Ward Sister, 5 staff nurses and 1 auxiliary. Of the staff nurses, one was on rotation to nights and one was usually on days off/annual leave. The ward had from 4 to 7 students, usually at least 5. It was unusual for the ward to have a third year student; there were normally 2 second years (in their first surgical rotation) and 3 first years. The number of staff assigned to each shift varied with the availability of students but usual staffing was 4 nurses on the early shift and 3 on the late shift. One of the nurses on each shift was a staff nurse or the Ward Sister. In addition, there was sometimes a nursing assistant or orderly.

[5] The early shift runs from 7:30 a.m. to 3:45 p.m. and the late shift from 1:00 p.m. to 9:00 p.m. Night staff are on the ward from 8:30 p.m. until 8:00 a.m. the next morning.

[6] 'Off-duty' is the staffing hour sheet that indicates the allocation of nurses to each of the 14 early and late shifts in a week.

[7] A number of these may be 'day cases', people who are admitted in the morning, have their procedure, recover on the ward and are discharged home in the evening.

6

Practising nursing

INTRODUCTION

The discussion so far has revealed experience and practice to be contextual and relational, forming and being formed by specific situations in particular times and places. When the Sisters' everyday practices are examined more closely, a process of practising is discerned. This process — of noticing, understanding and acting — is evident in the relational and contextual nature of the Sisters' practices. Although noticing, understanding and acting can be differentiated conceptually, in practice they are not so neatly segmented. Rather, they are inextricably intertwined in a non-linear, non-sequential process. The qualitative character of this process seems to contribute to the complex, multifaceted, goal-directed and patient-centred nature of the Sisters' practice. Arising from the discussion of this process are implications for the way in which we understand the nature of expertise in nursing practice.

NOTICING, UNDERSTANDING AND ACTING

Three distinct, yet inextricably intertwined processes characterize how the Sisters relate through their caring practices to their patients and to the ward. They are noticing, understanding and acting (Figure 6.1). Noticing is more than seeing, hearing or assessing: it is a process of interpretation. Understanding is more than a surface knowing or recognition: it is a deep comprehension of meanings inherent in a situation. And acting goes beyond mere behaviour or deployment of skills: it is practising in a concrete situation.

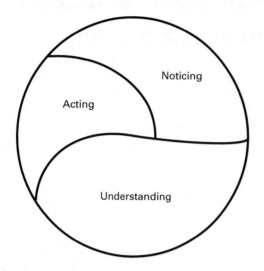

Figure 6.1   Noticing, understanding, acting

Through their involved stance in the situation, the Sisters notice salient features, understand their meaning and act, making the ward work; caring for the patient. Sr Aitkin notices Betty's jeans, understands what they mean in terms of her readiness to begin to be 'normal' again in social situations, and acts by 'pushing', encouraging her to go to the pub's bar. As she helps him to prepare for the upcoming surgery, Sr Ellis notices the character of Mr Peet's protestations, understands, has a feeling that he is frightened and unsure, and acts, explaining 'from the beginning'. Sr Baxter notices a student's 'wee delay' in responding to her suggestion that she takes out a patient's central line; she understands the delay to be a sign of a lack of knowledge and confidence and she acts, arranging for the student to observe the procedure again (Int. 2-3: 18). Noticing is made possible through the Sisters' experiences in previous, similar situations, which have made understanding possible.

Noticing and understanding are inextricably bound to the present context, as action occurs in an ongoing, concrete situation. Noticing and understanding are made possible by action. Sr Aitkin is with Betty on the ward, watching how she prepares herself, noticing and understanding the meanings of her preparations. Sr Ellis is present with Mr Peet, understanding where he is in relation to preparing for a major loss. Sr Jarvis

and Sr Baxter continually experience being with students on the ward, understanding how they learn to do procedures and noticing what happens to the student and the patient when they are inadequately prepared. How the Sisters go about caring for patients through making the ward work is an active, interpretative process. Even though they are intertwined in practice, noticing, understanding and acting are separated here for the purposes of discussion.

Noticing

When Sisters notice aspects of a situation, they are paying attention to some things more than to others. They interpret the situation and identify what is salient, what stands out to them. The Sisters often notice more particularly and widely: what is salient to the Sisters is often overlooked by less experienced nurses. In noticing, the Sisters pick out what is meaningful and in doing so, interpret something *as* something. Noticing is grounded in their understanding of the situation and occurs in the flow of action. The Sisters' involvement in situations with patients and others in the ward sets up the opportunity to notice; they are attuned to what is going on about them.

Noticing the 'little things'

In many instances, what the Sisters notice are 'little things', which may be small, but are not unimportant.[1] Sr Aitkin notices when Mrs Davies begins to take notice of something beyond herself.

Sr Aitkin: [...] Freddy was a very nice budgie actually. [...] I'm quite sure [he] sensed when Mabel wasn't very well. That was the mystery. On the day she went to theatre he was very quiet. Normally he was chirp chirp chirp.
     But Mrs Davies who was opposite said, 'I will talk to Freddy'. She said, 'Bring Freddy across to me'. And she couldn't really see very well. [...] And she talked to Freddy the whole of the morning. And Freddy responded quite well to her. But she was concerned for Mabel. She was concerned that Freddy was worried about... I mean I know that maybe it sounds trivial, but to me this has got importance. Mrs Davies was caring about somebody else. (Int. 1-1: 18)

An action which may have been considered trivial and its importance gone unnoticed by others, is salient for Sr Aitkin. She notices Mrs Davies' action and understands its meaning in relation to her recovery. She knows that in illness a person's world centres on themselves; as they recover, they can look outward and care for others. This was a sign of a step forward. Sr Aitkin's understanding of recovery and her knowledge of Mrs Davies, gives her an understanding of the situation and enables her to notice the significance of this action.

It is not only specific actions which the Sisters notice. They also notice how patients are: the expressions on their faces and in their postures. They notice what is said and what is not said, along with how it is said. Sr Ellis notices how Mr Peet responds during their conversations; she notices the pattern of the conversation, what is hidden by his protests and goes on to reveal and deal with his concerns. Sr Dunn watches the patients' faces closely when she dresses their wounds, noticing any sign of pain and adjusting her touch in response to what she senses. The Sisters are attuned to normal sounds and smells and notice small deviations from normal. They notice when someone's breathing pattern is changing; they notice small changes in the smell of wounds. When I noted her seemingly automatic smelling of the packing which she removed from wounds, Sr Ellis expressed surprise,

'I smell everything, don't you? I can tell by the smell of a dressing, what antibiotic to use. :: But it's not scientific :: I can smell on people's breath, that they have cancer and will need a laryngectomy :: Yes, there's a cancer smell.' (W5D2: 11)

As the Sisters develop expertise, the skill of their bodies gives them access to a situation with less effort and increased sensitivity (Benner & Tanner 1987). They become increasingly able to notice fine variations. Rather than being able to name specific components of what they notice, they notice wholes and discrepancies in those wholes — the smell of cancer on a person's breath, the feel of a circulation-impaired foot, the comportment of a patient in pain.

The Sisters have a finely-tuned sense of the normal pattern of patient recovery in relation to the workflow of the day and notice when things are not as expected. One morning, Sr Inglis notices the empty bed of a man who should not be walking on his infected foot. She finds him in the bathroom, reminds him he should not be up on his foot, and then has a quiet word with the orderly who got him up (W9D2-1: 11). The Sisters expect to see a certain pattern and timing of care and activity with each patient. When there is a variation, the Sisters notice; it signals action to be taken.

The Sisters' ability to notice more broadly yet particularly than less experienced nurses is evident when they notice salient features of the work of the ward. On her first day back from holiday, Sr Calder takes out a young man's intravenous cannula, 2 days after it could have come out. Nurses giving him bed baths during those 2 days had not taken it out, nor sought permission to take it out.

Sr Calder: But my professional instinct tells me he doesn't need that in. OK. He needed it when he was having intravenous antibiotics. He doesn't need it in; take it out. (Int. 3-3: 28)

When Sr Calder notices the intravenous cannula, she makes linkages: she remembers where he is in the course of treatment, that he is recovering and no longer needs intravenous antibiotics. The meaning of the intravenous cannula at this time for her is that it is an oversight in care. Her confidence in her judgement is such that it is now 'professional instinct'. Noticing prompts actions.

Throughout their workday, the Sisters notice the flow of work, gaps in the care of patients, how nurses are coping with their workload, how doctors are practising, how services are working and the feel of the ward atmosphere. They notice patterns and subtle changes or gaps in patterns, and respond to them. Noticing is holistic and situational.

Noticing all the time

The Sisters talk about looking and seeing or picking things up. 'You can stand at the nurses' station and look around and pick things up' (Int. 9-3: 51). They notice through the action of looking. 'But you know, I can just sort of walk around and have a look and [...] I know, like at a glance. But that's something that you just, you're looking out of practice' (Int. 5-3: 20). Sr Ellis looks 'out of practice'. She understands what she is seeing, even when it is 'at a glance'. Through their experience, the Sisters have come to be able to 'read a situation' (N Diekelmann, personal communication, 1990) and immediately focus on the problematic areas.

Furthermore, even when they are not actively seeking, the Sisters are noticing. 'You're always aware. You can always hear' (Int. 2-3: 24). As she is passing the treatment room on her medication rounds, Sr Ellis hears a 12-year-old boy crying as the doctor is cleaning his nose, a routine procedure. The other nurses, sitting near the room, do not notice. Sr Ellis asks one to go to him and brings the boy's distress to their attention, 'It's awful at that age. He's young' (W5D2-2: 10). As they do not seem to be hearing, Sr Ellis interprets the meaning of the boy's distress and his need for comfort. The Sisters are attuned to the normal sounds of patients and of the ward.

It is about 1120. Sr Grant says to me that at about 1130 or 1200, everything goes quiet on the ward. 'Everyone looks washed and their beds are made. If that doesn't happen and we don't hear that time, I know we're having a bad day.' (W7D2: 13)

They notice when the normal sounds and sights of the ward change and interpret their meaning. Being attuned comes from experience and from being involved in the practice situation.

Promoting noticing

The Sisters promote noticing in their interactions with students. With a patient who is bleeding postoperatively, Sr Jarvis cues the student about what to keep 'a very close eye' on (Int. 10-2: 21). Sr Calder tells the students to compare the similar responses of two patients to their different operations (W3D2: 4). Sr Inglis asks directly, 'He has a heparin pump. Do you know why?' (W9D1: 17). She goes on to tell about this patient's particular problems with anticoagulant regulation. The Ward Sisters not only give factual information, they interpret the patients' conditions, cueing junior nurses about the salient features of the patients and

their situation. They are helping the junior nurses learn how to notice, to pick up and to interpret.

Understanding

A Sister already has an understanding of any situation, a stance or prejudgement from which she interprets actions and meanings. She has, in Gadamer's words, 'a horizon of understanding' (Gadamer 1975). This horizon has been formed in the Sisters' previous experiences and is how the resource of experience shows itself in current situations. Sr Jarvis understands postoperative haematuria as normal or abnormal depending upon its nature and the specific context. Sr Baxter chooses to 'go with' a patient or not from her understanding of the particular patient and his needs at that time.

Understanding includes sharing background meanings: sharing meanings of being a patient and a nurse; sharing cultural meanings of language, facial expressions, and human experience. Understanding is not just knowing facts about something. It includes knowing the meanings inherent in particular situations. Sr Dunn, who routinely cares for patients with chronic chest wounds who have empyema tubes replaced weekly, knows more than simply how to insert an empyema tube skilfully. She has a broader and deeper knowledge: of the situation in which patients have empyema tubes inserted, of the meaning for the patient of a chronic wound, and of what it means to be an outpatient for a long period of time. Her understanding includes knowing what to look for in the patient's countenance and how to respond to what she sees there. It comes from knowing the patient in this instance in time, knowing the patient's history as well as having a shared history of previous encounters. Sr Dunn's interpretation of the situation, interpretation of the person's response, interpretation of the physical ease or resistance of the tube as it is inserted, are all grounded in her understanding of the situation she is in with the patient. Understanding comes from the past, is grounded in the present, but is geared towards the future.

Understanding enables noticing

Understanding makes it possible for the Sister to have a non-reflective, direct grasp of the situation. It enables noticing. With experience, the Sisters come to understand what counts as a 'usual' or 'normal' course of recovery and what patients are like on successive postoperative days. Their understanding enables them to notice when patients do not follow an expected or usual pattern. It alerts them to problems. A patient with 'swinging' fever, whose breathing is 'not quite clear' 2 days after nasal surgery is described by Sr Fraser as someone who is 'brewing an infection' or perhaps has a septal haematoma. She 'doesn't look right' (Int. 6-3: 2–3). From their extensive experience of patients who do 'look right', the Sisters have a complex understanding of what is normal, they notice slight deviations and understand what might underly the altered pattern of recovery.

In many situations, the Sisters' understandings are confirmed, enhanced or augmented. However, such confirmation does not seem to have led to rigidity in their practice. The Sisters encounter new situations flexibly and reflexively. They seem to consider their practice to be always open to question, and situations to be open to alternative understandings. As noticing comes from understanding in certain ways, some meanings may be overlooked in situations. Sr Hanna tells of a situation which she failed to interpret correctly. It concerned a woman who came into the ward following what might have been an illegal abortion.

Sr Hanna: [Now] If they've got pelvic inflammatory disease then it's usually, due to the coil or the fact that they've had a termination of pregnancy and they've got retained products or something like that. [. . .]
I can remember as a student nurse working in Ward G and it was the time of illegal abortions. [. . .] And you were aware of things like that all the time. 9 out of 10 ladies that presented themselves on a waiting night to your ward, it was because of an illegal abortion. [. . .] While I've been here as a Sister, it's something that is a way back, back at the back of your mind. [. . .] Unless there's other circumstances that bring it forward to your mind. [. . .] It's not something that immediately springs to mind when you have a lady in with pelvic inflammatory disease. While it was

the first thing you thought of when someone came in with bleeding and temperature and everything. 20 years ago you immediately thought, 'Oh this is an illegal abortion'. (Int. 8-2: 18–20)

Because there has been only one or two such cases in the last 5 years, Sr Hanna's understanding of a woman presenting herself with those symptoms has changed. Although her knowledge about illegal abortion as a possibility has been at the back of her mind since the legalization of abortion she has not been called upon to think along these lines. This situation has stimulated her to reconsider the understanding on which she bases her assessment of these patients – how she notices them; it reminds her to 'think along certain lines' so she does not mis-assess such women in the future. In a significant sense, the Sisters are in dialogue, so to speak, with their practice. They are open to new ways of understanding, acting and noticing.

Understanding informs acting

Understanding is always in a situation and it shows itself in practice. It informs differing actions. On rounds with the night nurses at 9:00 p.m. before she goes home, Sr Ellis goes to talk with 5-year-old Greg's mother who is sitting on the next bed, watching television. The side rails are down on the lowered bed as Greg sleeps. Sr Ellis does not pull them up. However, the night nurse comes into the room and puts them up immediately, waking the child. She does not look at Greg or his mother; turns and goes out of the room. Sr Ellis and the night nurse notice different things as they go into the room. Their understanding of the situation is differently informed (W5D4: 20). Sr Ellis says of her understanding, 'If there was a need Janet [the assigned nurse on the late shift] would have had them up. She's been an enrolled nurse for 2 years. She's not a novice' (W5D5: 2). Sr Ellis brings to her understanding of the immediate situation, her knowledge of the care the boy would have received from his assigned nurse. She does not notice anything 'out of the ordinary' as she goes into the room. In her understanding of the situation, Sr Ellis does not institute 'protective' measures for the boy, she spends her time in the room asking his mother if she needs anything and how she is finding her son. The night nurse, on the other hand, does not take into account these same understandings; she notices differently and her action stems from a different and perhaps less informed understanding.

Knowledge in understanding

Both practical know-how and theoretical knowledge inform understanding. In much of the Sisters' practice, it is impossible to identify them separately. When the Sisters teach students, however, their theoretical knowledge becomes more apparent. Knowledge of pressure and its practical implications informs Sr Grant's approach as she guides a student through the procedure of removing a central venous pressure catheter.

Sr Grant goes to help Nurse Elias, a third-year student, take out Mr Baker's CVP. Sr Grant tells Nurse Elias, 'If it is a positive CVP it means that the pressure in there (pointing to his chest) is less than the air. If the CVP is negative, the pressure of the air is greater. What position should he be in if it is negative, to avoid having an air embolism?' Nurse Elias: 'Sitting?' 'No, that would decrease the pressure in the chest.' Nurse Elias: 'Head further down.' 'Yes.' Sr Grant then supervises as Nurse Elias takes it out. [. . .] As Nurse Elias takes it out, Sr Grant says, 'Give it traction, steady traction, pulling up. :: [. . .] Sr Grant repeats at the end of the procedure that the most important thing to remember is to have Mr Baker in a flat position. (W7D5: 16)

Sr Grant does not go into the details of pressure in the chest, but reminds Nurse Elias of the relationship of posture to pressure and of the reading of the central line to air pressure. Although theoretical principles inform her instruction, she focuses on the practical knowledge of the procedure. Sr Grant's understanding of central lines and their removal is neither solely theoretical nor practical. An admixture of theoretical knowledge and practical know-how shows in her practice.

Understanding also stems from the Sisters knowing themselves as human beings and through relating to patients as fellow human beings. When Sr Baxter suggests to a 20-year-old appendectomy patient, who is reluctant to move, that she wash her hair whilst showering, the suggestion comes from her own understanding.

Sr Baxter: [. . .] You know yourself if you're not feeling 100%, and you've been in bed for a few days, and you haven't felt up to the mark. What do you do? You like to have a bath and wash your hair and you feel so much better. You don't have to do anything else. Change your nightie. And you feel so much better. And that probably stems from . . . you and feelings that you feel yourself when you're unwell. (Int. 2-2: 20)

Sr Baxter calls on her own knowledge of the little things in normal life, things that make you feel better, to help a patient feel better in herself, to help her 'over the hump'. The Sisters do not stand outside the situation as onlooking, distanced professionals but are involved with the patient in the situation as persons, and as nurses who can call upon their own understanding of being human.[2]

Understanding in context

Understanding is both formed in a context and shows itself in a context. This is particularly evident when the Sisters talk about knowing the patients. As much as the Sisters understand the patients as people and fellow human beings, they recognize that they only know the patient as a patient in hospital, and that he or she may be 'a different person' outside this immediate context.

Sr Ellis: . . . You know unfortunately we didn't know Mr Peet . . . before. We hadn't met him before his operation. Particularly because he'd had the trachy in-between times. But we felt in that day we got to know him fairly well. But having said that in 2 weeks time you could see a completely different Mr Peet, which might be the real one, you know. (Int. 5-3: 10)

The Sisters know patients as people who are in the midst of illness and hospitalization. As patients are on the ward for a limited time, they know them in a very specific temporal context. However, within the limits and opportunities afforded by the context, the Sisters know the patients well (MacLeod 1993). Occasionally, a patient can even become 'an old friend' (Int. 8-1:

4) or 'great buddies' (Int. 9-1: 11), but these closer relationships are still between patient and nurse; they remain contextual. Understanding the patients and the work of the ward is knowing in and of a context.

Sharing understanding

Understanding is largely taken-for-granted and tacit (Polanyi [1958]1962). It comes forth in practice, often not coming into awareness. Understanding cannot be broken down into discrete pieces or be frozen in time. The flow of the Sisters' practice reveals understanding to be whole and fluid. Frequently, understanding and the noticing which arises from it, are hidden, not only from the Sister, but also from the observer of her practice.

When we are at Mr Ferry's bed, Sr Calder asks him if he would like to go home today, that she thought he just might if the doctors felt he was ready. She asks him whether he could get transportation. He says no, that his wife could come in, but he would have to go by taxi. Sr Calder says, 'Yes, a taxi. Where do you live?' He says, 'Just across the Common'. Sr Calder says, 'Fine' and moves on. I ask him, 'What floor does he live on?' (Sr Calder makes a face at me) He says he has a second floor flat. (Sr Calder doesn't say anything and just moves on — she isn't concerned.)
At the time, the thought went through my mind that Sr Calder may not have wanted to hold up the discharge, and wasn't concerned about his crutch walking, but I wondered why she didn't have the physio check him out on the stairs (although I knew that physios had to be specially consulted that day and it might have been difficult). (W3D2: 7)
[Later at coffee] I ask her about her decision about Mr Ferry and why she did not pursue the crutches and the fact that he lived on the second floor. She says that she didn't even have it in the back of her mind until I asked the question, and then his managing on the stairs came to the front of her mind. Sr Calder replied: 'I worked my way backwards', to when he came in. He came in on crutches and had been on them at home. So he would have had to have managed the stairs and would have had the physio teach him how to manage stairs.
'Because that wasn't a concern at all', she said, 'I didn't pursue it'. Had I not mentioned it, it would not have come to her mind at all. Not because she overlooked it, but because it didn't need to be there, particularly as she saw him walk [on crutches] the previous evening. She noted then how well he did ('You have this aced'). (W3D2: 10)

Sr Calder and I come to this situation with different understanding. When talking to Mr Ferry, I have forgotten about his solid success on crutches. Thinking that stairs should always be considered in such a discharge conversation, I assume it has been overlooked. Sr Calder, however, has already picked up on Mr Ferry's ability to use crutches, 'working [her] way back' to when he came in. She understands Mr Ferry to be a person who is capable of managing on crutches where he lives. As she interprets his needs for assistance in discharge, 'that wasn't a concern at all'. It is not to say Sr Calder overlooks this aspect of Mr Ferry's care, rather her understanding of him already incorporates it. She does not pick up anything in the conversation or from his actions in hospital to change it, to bring this concern to the 'front of her mind'. Her understanding is not readily apparent to me, and I misconstrue it.

Misconstrual of their practices by less experienced nurses and the frustration it provokes was described by several of the Sisters. It is like the tip of an iceberg. The contexts of understanding within which the Sisters operate are complex; they are easy to ignore or overlook when individual actions are all that is evident.

One consequence of having extensive understanding of patterns of activity and of taking knowledge for granted, is that such knowledge often cannot be easily expressed. However, just because it is difficult to put into words does not mean that understanding is absent.

Andrew [a 24-year-old athletic looking man] is up on crutches with the physio. Sr Calder watches him walk down the hall, out the door and towards the stairs. 'He's away.' I ask her how she knows. 'Look at him — just look at him — he's young — just look.' I have to agree. A few minutes later, [. . .] the physio comes back with Andrew. She asks, 'Was Andrew allowed to go home when he was safe to go?' Sr Calder: 'Mnhmn'. Physio: 'He's safe'. (W3D3: 7)

Describing a pattern, a whole, is not easy when our usual ways of describing are through properties or attributes. In saying 'He's away', Sr Calder is recognizing Andrew's ability on crutches. She sees his confidence in the whole of how he moves. She knows his recovery pattern so far and can project what it may continue to be. 'He's young' reflects her understanding of his capacity and energy to become mobile and 'safe to go'. Sr Calder does not describe the parts to me, she invites me to use my powers of recognition of patterns and my commonsense. 'I have to agree.' By looking, really looking and noticing, grounded in my understanding of how people are and move, I join her in understanding.

When Sisters work alongside junior nurses, they frequently read situations together. It helps the junior nurses to develop their skills in noticing and also helps them towards new understandings. Importantly, it helps junior nurses to develop confidence in their abilities to understand situations and the context of human actions. Sisters sometimes ask patients' families to read the situation of recovery with them. Reading situations together allows the Sister and family to share understandings with the effect that both gain new insights and have the opportunity to notice differently. It creates a human sharing and a bond of common understanding.

Acting: practising nursing

Although acting comes third in this discussion, noticing and understanding have emerged out of ongoing action, the practice of surgical nursing. In Chapter 5, the Sisters' practice was detailed. This section extends that discussion by exploring several key ingredients. The first is involvement, how the Sisters' care and concern enables their practice with their patients in everyday work situations. Second is how the Sisters maintain a flexible stance, changing their practice to suit the specific situation. Third is the confidence they have in their practice and the sureness and authority which stems from it. Although these ingredients are identified for the purposes of discussion, they are inseparable from the Sisters' ongoing practice.

Practising from an involved stance

The Sisters can be said to be involved in and of the situation. Although involvement, in common usage, can mean 'entangled' or 'rolled up in', the Sisters are not involved in that way. Rather, they are involved in the sense of being 'implicitly contained' in the situation. In their caring practices, the Sisters are with the person, where the person is, both in space and time. They do not stand outside as onlookers, nor are they only there in body with their minds elsewhere. Being involved is understood to be a caring and 'concernful' stance (Heidegger 1962, Benner & Wrubel 1989) from which the Sisters practise.

This stance neither drips with emotion, nor is it instrumental. It simply stems from the commitment of the Sister to care for people.

Sr Dunn: .... I think you feel something inside you for these, for people who are are ill and who need help, not in a 'I feel so sorry for you' attitude or anything like that. I think you just feel that you want to help these people. And if there's anything you can do that will make them better or ... make their life better you would like to be part of that. (Int. 4-2: 44–45)

This sentiment is aptly echoed by Altschul (1979) as she writes:

We nurses choose to commit ourselves to the sick, the helpless, the incompetent, not with any sentimentality or with any ulterior motive of bringing greater glory to ourselves, but simply because we have chosen an existence in which concern for the welfare of these people gives us a purpose in life. (p 125)

This caring stance infuses the Sisters' everyday work. It is not only the patients and the ward which matter, the Sisters also care about the system within which they work.

Sr Aitkin gives at report: 'Morag :: from the renal unit [...] is to have Dextrose 10% and insulin and potassium, to keep her potassium levels as normal as possible at 20 ml/hour :: It is to go in at 0800 :: There's no point at putting it in at 0800, as the renal Registrar is coming here to take blood for her potassium levels. It will give her the wrong reading :: We'll put it up after she comes'.

The Registrar comes up at 0835 and takes the blood. Sr Aitkin puts up the solution about 0900 [. . .] At 0930, the Registrar phones saying that the potassium levels are high and the infusion needs to be changed to Dextrose 5% with no potassium and insulin at 10 ml/hour. Sr Aitkin grumbles about the cost to the health service and the inefficiency of it. (W1D2-2: 5)

Sr Aitkin anticipates the doctor's actions and coordinates the intravenous infusion on the basis of that anticipation. When the doctor changes the order, Sr Aitkin is not only concerned about wasted efforts, but also about the cost to the health service. It is not unusual to hear the Sisters say, turning off a light or conserving supplies, 'We'll save some money for the NHS'. The organization matters.

The Sisters' involvement shows itself in their practice, their understanding and their capacity to notice. Their concerned, involved stance enables them to notice meaningful aspects and possibilities inherent in the situation. Through their involvement they understand more deeply and broadly. Having said that, when an approach is not working well, or a problem is not amenable to the current solution, the Sisters 'take a backward step and reassess the situation' and 'find another way of dealing with it' (Int. 8-1: 5). In so doing, they gain a different perspective, notice differently, or access a different understanding. This stepping backward is not stepping aside. It is remaining *with* the situation, while finding another way of being in it.

Practising flexibly

The Sisters practise in a flexible way, tailoring their care to the particular person and situation. This flexibility is possible because they have a very clear sense of their 'ends-in-view' (Dewey 1925), helping patients towards recovery through both direct action and making the ward work. Their repertoire of experiences and skills have enabled them to notice and understand the alternative paths towards these ends-in-view which exist in any particular situation. Thus, the Sisters have complex goals for seemingly simple

endeavours. What appears to be delivering breakfasts or giving out medications encompasses a brief yet detailed assessment of the patients. The Sisters consistently respond to the inherent possibilities in the situation and tailor their practices to take advantage of them.

Far from being instrumental or mechanical, the Sisters' practices are purposive. The timing and pacing of Sr Ellis' intervention to 'protect' Dr Campbell as he gives a family bad news turns a simple practice of monitoring and supporting into something that is unique to that particular situation and the people in it. Sr Inglis' system of ensuring that wounds are checked is more than a simple routine. It helps to ensure a certain quality of care. The intentional nature of the Sisters' interventions take such practices from the realm of task or rote activities into the realm of thoughtful practice (Glass 1983). Rather than the Sisters' focus being on the task, the focus is on the end-in-view and on the goals for the situation in that particular point in time. It is by understanding the possibilities inherent in the situations, and by understanding that there are many avenues which will lead to their ends-in-view that the Sisters are able to practise flexibly.

The Sisters' knowledge and understanding allows them to 'break the rules' in practice. They know when and how they can be flexible to suit the needs of the patients and the ward. Sr Grant breaks her own rules about admitting patients when flexibility is called for (Int. 7-3: 10–11). She knows when she can be flexible yet still maintain her authority and clear role distinction. Sr Aitkin tells the student to stop taking a dying woman's temperature. 'We're not going to treat her with antibiotics :: If you take it you just worry about it' (W1D2-1: 17). She alters the routine for the patient's comfort; it also serves to focus the student's attention on the patient. When the Sisters break the rules it is for the patient. However, when the rules are broken or knowledge is adapted in practice, the formal knowledge is not discarded. It is transformed into something which suits the situation. Sr Dunn tells about how she changes the procedure of inserting an empyema tube from a sterile procedure to a clean one.

Sr Dunn: [. . .] Sometimes I pick up the tube and I haven't got gloves on. Because I can't work, sticking that pin on. I try to be very careful and not touch anything. [. . .] You just have to use your own judgement. And you don't go and do things completely wrong. [. . .] I've probably adapted doing these dressings the way I find it easier for the patients. (Int. 4-3: 19–21)

Sr Dunn maintains the principles of asepsis as much as she can, 'you don't go and do things completely wrong', but centrally, she adapts it for the patients. As the patients need these tubes changed weekly over a long period of time, she adapts her practice to find a way in which she can keep the procedure as clean as possible, yet as comfortable as possible for the patients. The Sisters shape their practice for the patients and the situation. 'Your practice adapts continually' (Int. 7-1: 14). Just as the Sisters' understanding remains open to change, so does their practice.

Practising confidently

The Sisters have confidence and a sureness in their practice. They take their confidence for granted; it is an essential constituent of their practice. A strong indicator of that confidence is that none of the Sisters takes extensive notes about the patients, even though some deal with up to 50 patients in a day. Some of the Sisters take occasional notes about things to do for patients as they go on rounds. One writes reminders to herself in a notebook about administrative details, for example to telephone about getting blinds repaired. But importantly, even though some take notes, none refers to them except after the fact, or as a check to see that all the tasks have been done. They remember an extraordinary amount of information about patients, their conditions and their progress. How they developed this skill is discussed in the next chapter, but here Sr Jarvis tells what it means to her to have this skill.

Sr Jarvis: I feel it is nice to be able to be seen to know everybody and know what's happening without

having to constantly refer to notes. I realize not everybody could work it like this, but I'm fortunate that I can. I don't like to see nurses, whatever grade they are, forever having to refer back to their bit of paper to remember who that patient is and what's wrong with them. I feel being able to go around, as I do on ward rounds, without having to constantly refer back and write things down gives that air of confidence and knowledge in what's happening. And also makes the patient see that the nurse knows who they are. They don't need to look up the notebook to see which bed they're in so, 'All right that must be her'. 'Oh that's what's wrong with her. All right, yes. I remember now.' You know. So I think that's why I like being able to do it. (Int. 10-3: 20)

Their confidence is enabling. When the Sisters are confident, other nurses and patients have confidence in them. 'It's just they can trust someone who has a bit of confidence in themselves' (W5D2-1: 6). Confidence plays a large role in how the Sisters notice, understand and act. Confident in their ability to understand and manage certain situations, the Ward Sisters are able to attend to concerns beyond the immediate situation. They notice more broadly. It is a key to their being able to manage the tension between attending to one patient and attending to all in the ward. Having confidence in themselves, the Sisters can be more flexible. When they 'can have confidence in others' (Int. 5-3: 20) they can delegate authority. And importantly, the 'confidence of experience' (Int. 5-3: 26) enables the Sisters to break the rules and tailor their practices to the situation. Confidence is crucial to the Sisters' effectiveness, authority and practice. 'It comes with experience' (W5D2-1: 6).

The Sisters' confidence, however, presents something of a paradox. The Sisters continually keep their practice open to question, yet their confidence bespeaks certainty. Certainty, in a milieu which is notoriously uncertain and changing can become dogmatic and dysfunctional, precluding openness (Katz 1988). However, this does not seem to be the case for the Sisters. The Sisters' confidence does not stem from the knowledge which labels and explains, rather it is interlinked with a knowing-in-practice which continually begs the question (Barker 1989).

A QUESTION OF PRACTISING EXPERTLY

Questions of expertise have repeatedly surfaced in this research. Are the Sisters expert surgical nurses? Does their practice exemplify expert practice? The study did not set out to address these questions, but they have arisen and have persisted. It may be helpful here to address them insofar as they can be addressed through the interviews and observations of practice.

An expert or practising expertly?

When I first sought nurses to participate in the study, I asked for 'experienced, excellent nurses'. I was seeking nurses who had benefited from their experience. The notion of an 'expert' nurse was not a comfortable nor familiar one within the nursing milieu in Scotland. However, the nursing administrators who were approached had no difficulty identifying nurses who were experienced and excellent, and who met the criteria for the study. These criteria are consistent with those used by Benner (1984) to identify experienced nurses who were 'recognized for their expertise' (p 14). Although Benner goes on to describe these experienced nurses as 'expert clinicians' (Benner 1984, Benner & Wrubel 1989, Benner et al 1992), that step has not been taken in this study for two reasons. The first concerns the focus of the study and the second relates to the difficulty in ascertaining what constitutes expertise.

The study centres on the Sisters as they practise and experience, not on them as individuals outwith particular situations. Indeed, it has shown nursing practice and experience to be relational and contextual. It means that nurses cannot be deemed to be experts in isolation from the very specific and particular situations in which they practise. This study supports the use of 'expert' as an adjective, describing practice, or more preferably as an adverb, describing practising, as opposed to using 'expert' as a noun to name a person. Whilst the Dreyfus Model of Skill Acquisition (Dreyfus & Dreyfus 1986), and

Benner's (1984, Benner et al 1992) application of it to nursing emphasize the contextual nature of expertise, both Dreyfus & Dreyfus and Benner move from this position to name individuals who exhibit expertise, 'experts'. This move may not be problematic in areas of endeavour which are relatively uniform, such as chess or car driving, but in areas such as nursing which are complex, highly variable and continually changing, there are more difficulties. The very fact that nurses care for people makes the situations in which they practise highly variable. Expertise in one situation with one person does not mean expertise in a similar situation with another. The Sisters may practise expertly, but labelling them 'experts' and thus implying they are experts in all areas of endeavour, is inconsistent with the notion that their practice is contextual and relational.

What constitutes expertise?

Although this study did not set out to distinguish expertise, the examination of the Sisters' practices and their process of practising has provided a wealth of insights into practising expertly. When the study began, the Dreyfus Model, with its emphasis on experience and practical knowledge, provided a useful touchstone for considering the practice of experienced nurses. The Sisters' practice has been interpreted as a process of noticing, understanding and acting. It is not an empty process, but one which is imbued with knowledge and skills in specific, concrete, particular situations. Thus, expertise as a descriptor of the quality of practice would need to concern both the process and the content of practice.

The Dreyfus Model is especially useful for directing our attention to the idea that expertise lies in practices and practical knowledge rather than in theoretical knowledge and traits or attributes of an individual. However, this study has illuminated some of the Dreyfus Model's limitations, particularly its emphasis on decision-making and its failure to address adequately the issue of the appropriateness of action for a situation.

Dreyfus & Dreyfus (1986) hold that a central characteristic of the expert is the use of intuition which shows itself in:

... involved skilled behaviour based on an accumulation of concrete experiences and the unconscious recognition of new situations as similar to whole remembered ones. (p 35)

The six key aspects of the expert's intuitive judgement: pattern recognition, similarity recognition, commonsense understanding, skilled know-how, a sense of salience and deliberative rationality (Dreyfus & Dreyfus 1986, Benner & Tanner 1987), are present in many of the Sisters' practices. However, there seems to be more to their practices than fluidly and intuitively approaching a task or making decisions.

Dreyfus & Dreyfus (1986) propose that a change from a distanced stance to an involved stance is a hallmark of moving from novice to expert. Following from this, it can be intimated that only skilled, expert practices can be deemed to be caring practices (Benner 1988, Benner & Wrubel 1989) as only proficient and expert performers are sufficiently engaged in the situation. However, being involved in a situation does not seem to be a simple or unitary phenomenon.

The Sisters' caring and involvement in patient situations do not seem to change with time. What changes is their ability to understand, notice and constructively practise in similar situations (Int. 4-2: 43). They become involved *differently*.

In their current practice, the Sisters often notice more widely yet focus more specifically and quickly on particular problem areas and the meaning for the patient. Less experienced nurses seem to be involved more narrowly and inwardly, being more concerned with their own performance and the work to be done in the present than with the patients and their concerns.

Sr Dunn: And as student nurse it was probably more important to me how I felt giving an injection, than it was how the patient felt. Again probably when I was a full time staff nurse it was probably more important to me how ...... at the end of a shift how the ward work had gone. Had I coped, had I managed. Whereas now [...] I think I am probably able to think more about, has the patient managed or has the patient coped. (Int. 4-1: 13)

This parallels Larsson's (1986) finding that when a teacher has taught for some time there is a change in his focus of attention 'from the teacher's own acts and/or planning, towards the pupil's acts and/or thinking'. This focus away from themselves may also explain, in part, why the Sisters found it easy for me to shadow them as they worked. Their focus was on the patient and the ward, not on their performance. Indeed, everyday physical and interpersonal activities are not mentioned in the interviews. They are taken for granted and the Sisters no longer 'see' them.

Unlike the Sisters, student nurses do not take technical procedures for granted. They focus directly upon them. This is seen among the learners in Melia's study (1983, 1987) who consider nursing care involving technical skills to be 'real nursing'. The inability of nurses who are still concerned with mastering technical skills to see beyond those skills could partly account for why learners and newly qualified nurses take the doctors as their reference point, often not recognizing the knowledge of experienced nurses until they are more experienced themselves (Int. 3-2: 2). The knowing of the experienced Sisters is more complex; both 'technical' and 'basic' skills are interconnected in their practices. The focus of their attention in a situation is commensurate with this knowing.

In addition to the issue of intuition and involvement in the situation — the process of practice — the study provides insight into the importance of the content of practice in expertise. It would seem that to be included in expert practice, a specific intervention, replete with its implicit goals, its timing and pacing, would need to be *a* (not necessarily *the*) right action for the particular patient or situation and the nurse at a particular moment in time. Whereas a less experienced nurse may approach activities with patients serially, the Sisters 'discover the possibilities inherent in the situation' (Benner & Wrubel 1989 p 396) and create complex goals which can be achieved simultaneously. This is the key to 'being organized'; the Sisters are able to do it in circumstances which are ever-changing. The goals and the Sisters' practices which achieve them are qualitatively different from those of junior nurses. They are expressed in part, through a recognition and appreciation of differences (N Diekelmann, personal communication, 1990) in contrast to the junior nurses' seeking of consistency. This study did not look at the outcome of the Sisters' practices with a view to assessing their appropriateness. However, it could be argued that such an assessment is implicit in the Sisters' practices as they continually monitor the effects of their actions and finely adjust them to the particular situation.

Thus, according to the Dreyfus Model, the Sisters could be said to be practising expertly in many situations. It would be misleading to suggest that they always practise expertly, or even with unqualified competence. Their practice simply was not addressed from an evaluative perspective. Having said that, it seems that this description of the practice of experienced nurses who have a reputation of being excellent clinical practitioners may offer some glimpses into practising expertly.

SUMMARY

This chapter has revealed that, for the Sisters, practising surgical nursing expertly is closely bound up with how they notice, understand and act in practice and the knowing embedded in their practice. They practise from a caring, concerned stance, being fully present in the situation and with people. Patients, the ward and the organization matter to them. They notice broadly and particularly. Their interpretation of the situation can be counted upon. The Sisters come to workday situations with solid backgrounds of understanding which inform and guide their interpretations in practice. Their understanding is situated and provisional. As the situation changes, so does their understanding. Dialogue characterizes their interactions; they are open with people and experiences in the ward. Flexibility, suiting their actions to the situation, is a hallmark of their practice. Like the expert nurses in Benner's (1984, Benner et al 1992) studies and in comparison to other nurses, in many situations the Sisters have a qualitatively different perception of the task environment. As well, they demonstrate a qualitative difference in their actions and skills. They approach many decisions and carry through their actions in an intuitive, fluid way. Finally, their knowing in practice is temporal, located solidly in the present situation, but drawing from the past and acting towards the possibilities of the future. The quality of their noticing, understanding and acting in their practice, as well as the timeliness, appropriateness and effectiveness of their practice, is how the Sisters may have become known as excellent, experienced nurses.

Notes

[1] For an extended discussion of 'It's the little things that count' see MacLeod (1994).

[2] See also Taylor (1994).

7

Becoming experienced

INTRODUCTION

A sense of the continuous interplay between experience and practice has clearly emerged from the Sisters' accounts and observations of their everyday practices. The Sisters have been shown to be 'experienced' Sisters who are experiencing all the time. Taking the process of practising to be one of noticing, understanding and acting, I have offered a glimpse into how experience and practice may be interconnected. In this chapter, I wish to take this discussion a step further by exploring the process of experiencing which enables the Sisters to become 'experienced'.

In Chapter 4, I suggested that experiencing, the moment-by-moment process of being, of acting in a situation, involves learning. Learning was said to accompany experiencing and to be an outgrowth of experience. We do not have a very good vocabulary to use when talking about the ongoing nature of experiencing. This is perhaps because it is something we are rarely aware of at the time and because it is always in a particular context. We may talk about our practices and our knowing but it seems that we commonly express our sense of the movement of experience by the term, *learning*.

The movement inherent in learning is reflected in the dictionary definition, which describes learning as an action of gaining, acquiring or becoming. The Sisters use the word 'learning' when they describe connections between past and present experiences and practices or when they talk about the meaning for them of particular experiences. The ways in which they describe learning reflect its situational and contextual nature and support Selman's (1988) contention that learning should be viewed as more than just being 'inside an individual's head'. Just as the Sisters' experiences are not private, but are public through language and practices (Taylor 1985), so too is their learning which is revealed in their everyday language and practices.

It is not uncommon in the adult learning literature to find a separation of experiences into 'learning experiences' and other experiences (cf. Brookfield 1986, Jarvis 1987a, 1987b). I have already pointed out the difficulties with this understanding of experience and have argued that a separation of learning experiences and other experiences could be considered spurious. After all, it seems that all of the Sisters' experience is potentially a resource in their ongoing experiencing. It is proposed here, that for the Sisters, learning is not only a result of some particularly meaningful experiences: it accompanies all experiencing.

Conceptions of learning which focus on internal, mental processes, albeit processes which may be influenced by the social milieu, reflect a dualistic view of the person in which the body and mind are considered to be separate entities (Brookfield 1986, Jarvis 1987a). This could account for why these theorists and others hold that some experiences involve the mind in learning while others may not. However, the Sisters' accounts and practices stand in stark contrast: they reveal experience and learning to be as much in the Sisters' fingertips as in their minds. They confirm the unity of the body and mind (Merleau-Ponty 1962, Heidegger 1962). Through their bodies, the Sisters have access to an understanding of which they are not always aware, and which they may not be able to describe. This perhaps reflects the intentionality and the memory which resides in habitual, bodily ways of knowing (Benner & Wrubel 1989, Schilder 1989). Further, it reflects the view that all our experiences are 'enfleshed' and that our body never 'forgets' (Duden 1991). If indeed our bodies never forget, then we gain experience in any situation in which we find ourselves, and therefore all situations are sources of learning.

Just as experience is an elusive and fluid phenomenon which does not lend itself to a uniform, simple description, so too is learning. As it would be misleading to dissect and simplify this complex and multifaceted phenomenon, I hope simply to point the way towards an understanding of how learning shows up in experiencing.

LEARNING ALL THE TIME

In talking about experience and learning Sr Inglis puts it simply yet profoundly, 'It's happening all the time' (Int. 9-3: 35). This almost throw-away remark points towards the contextual and relational nature of learning. Just as noticing, understanding and acting depict the process of practising, so they could be taken to describe the process of experiencing. Taking learning to depict the movement of experiencing, it could be said that learning encompasses changes in noticing, understanding and acting. In addition, learning is made possible by noticing, understanding and acting.

In Chapter 4, the range and variability of the Sisters' experiences were described and the majority were seen to be taken-for-granted ('bits and bobs') or 'resonant' experiences. Not surprisingly perhaps, the Sisters' learning parallels this. Whilst there are certainly instances in which the Sisters describe having sudden insight, the majority of the Sisters' references to learning use physical metaphors such as 'picking up' or 'absorbing'. These physical metaphors reveal learning which is gradual and sometimes imperceptible, though far from insignificant. They also reveal something of the fluid nature of learning, as new meanings are found in the juxtaposition of past experience and ongoing experiencing.

Learning as sudden insight

Gaining insight can be a sudden or a gradual process. Often sudden insights are part of 'watershed' experiences. In the following experience, Sr Aitkin has a flash of insight, she 'suddenly learnt' about her own practice.

Sr Aitkin: I think I can remember very well, maybe to the exact day, that I was put in my place by a staff nurse. Who I was very fond of and I think she was very fond of me. I [. . .] had a very busy 36-bedded female surgical ward and they were very busy this particular March. And I was on an early and I should have gone home, but I always like to finish my own work before I go home. [. . .] And I was very concerned for this girl because I knew she was going to be busy. She was just about to start her drugs. There were patients coming back from theatre and there were the suppers to get out. Although we had a very good domestic who would have done [. . .] anything for you.

And I said to the staff nurse, 'Would you like me to stay behind and help? Would you like me to do the suppers for you before I go?' And she turned to me and she said, 'Sister would you PLEASE go home. I can manage'. And I felt dreadful. I really did feel dreadful. And I thought, 'Oh my.' And it was like a slap in the face because we had a very good relationship [. . .]. And I thought, 'Oh dear'. [. . .]

I went [. . .] home. And [the girl I flatted out with] said, 'God you're late again'. [. . .] And I told her and I was actually quite upset about it. And she turned [laugh] and she said, 'Well she did the right thing'. And I thought, 'OH!! nobody wants me'. And then she said, 'But Jenny you've got to stand back and let these kids develop. You're not helping THEM'.

Although she said, 'Who do you think you're helping? Is it making you feel good that you're staying behind'. And yet she could see. She said, 'I can see what you want. You want your patients all right. You want them to have their supper at six o'clock. But it's not fair on the staff nurse because she can't plan her own evening if you're going to be there all the time to do it'. And they were both very right, VERY RIGHT. [. . .]

But I suddenly learnt well you can't just go on. (Int. 1-1: 30–32)

This sudden insight into her own practice comes for Sr Aitkin in the aftermath of an unexpected rebuke from a respected staff nurse. Her immediate experience of being 'put in my place' is reframed by her flatmate who helps Sr Aitkin understand the effects of not delegating fully. It is a milestone for Sr Aitkin in gaining an ability to broaden her focus of concern from purely the short-term needs of patients to the needs of staff and patients in the longer term. For her, it is a key in learning how to be a Ward Sister in a new way which is helpful both to her staff and herself. Sometimes, however, insights are not quite as abrupt, but come after a period of imperceptible change and may not be as emotionally charged.

After 9 months experience of being a Ward Sister, Sr Inglis notices one day '. . . I was no longer apprehensive . . .' and she learns she is comfortable in the job, '. . . I realized that I was home'. Such a realization transforms her confidence: 'Now I feel no matter what was thrown at me, I may not know about it but I could handle it' (Int. 9-3: 10). And with the confidence, her experience of being a Ward Sister is transformed. She is no longer anxious, but becomes 'expectant', and 'always prepared for something to happen' (Int. 9-3: 11).

Prompted by noticing a difference in their own understanding or feelings about a situation or their work, the Sisters realize that they have learned about their way of being a Ward Sister. They locate their learning in a particular time and place, but it may have stemmed from a single experience, or from experiences over several months. These times of sudden insights are occasionally referred to as 'turning points'. They are an identifiable point of change, when the Sisters' realization of alternative options or new ways of being, changes their practice.

Learning as 'having it instilled into us'

Learning in many situations is a more gradual and perhaps more passive process. Some of the Sisters spoke of nursing knowledge being 'dinned into us' (Int. 3-3: 25), or '. . . just bred into you' (Int. 1-1: 27) by ward sisters and tutors, particularly during the early stages of their training. Living up to expectations, 'having to do it' and wanting to do their best drove them. 'We had to do it. And we did it' (Int. 3-3: 25).

The knowledge they learned in this way (anatomy and physiology, the importance of working neatly or remembering patients' names) may not have been particularly meaningful at the time, but the Sisters have since recognized new meaning in it. Remembering patients' names was a skill developed early in training.

Sr Jarvis: . . . . I can remember as a student on night duty . . . One of the biggest worries on nights and it still exists for the students, is that the nursing officer is going to come into that ward at any time and ask you to do a ward round with them about the patients.

And you'd had report from whoever had been on and you'd written everybody's name down and their age and their diagnosis. And then you put it in your pocket and you'd got on with your routine of doing your temperatures and drug round and whatever else. And we used to then, if we had time after the patients had settled, sit and practise going round the ward in a set order.

Start at the 'left one' or whatever it was and reel off the patient's name and their age and their diagnosis, so that you learned it from memory. And it would throw you completely if they started the other side. [laugh] (Int. 10-3: 18–19)

Although the Sisters' skill of remembering patients begins early in training, it evolves and takes on new meaning over time, as Sr Jarvis explained in Chapter 6. The way of remembering is also transformed.

Sr Fraser: After a while, once I've got the patients in my head and I know who THEY are, I can monitor the changes that way. I can do it mentally, without writing it down. (Int. 6-3: 9)

A broader understanding of the patient and changed responsibilities have brought both new relevance to remembering patients and changes in their care. The Sisters' way of remembering has changed from learning by rote and for the benefit of someone else, to learning 'who *they* are', because it enables them to give better care. Thus it moves, from the instilling of the early years of training, to a more active way of learning as the Sisters come to understand the value and meaning of the skill differently with time.

Learning as absorbing

While 'having it instilled into us' describes a process in which the Sisters learn despite themselves to suit the requirements of an authority figure, 'learning as absorbing' describes a perhaps less obvious process of learning by example. Sr Grant notes how staff nurses, 'particularly if they're new to their role, will absorb everything you do, and your style to a certain extent' (Int. 7-3: 19). Bandura (1977) calls this absorption, 'modelling'. As Polanyi ([1958]1962) contends, this kind of uncritical imitation is necessary, particularly when much of the knowing which is to be learned cannot be specified in detail nor transmitted by prescription.

To learn by example is to submit to authority. You follow your master because you trust his manner of doing things even when you cannot analyze and account in detail for its effectiveness. By watching the master and emulating his efforts in the presence of his example, the apprentice unconsciously picks up the rules of the art, including those which are not explicitly known to the master himself. These hidden rules can be assimilated only by a person who surrenders himself to that extent uncritically to the imitation of another. (p 53)

However, not everything about a person is absorbed. The Sisters also talk about ward sisters with less endearing qualities who, nevertheless, greatly influenced them. Although an influential ward sister had a 'very, very domineering manner', Sr Hanna admired other aspects of how she worked, and took away from her 'an ability ... to cope with anything at my work regardless of my home circumstances' (Int. 8-3: 27). The qualities absorbed from working with a ward sister would sometimes be cast in a new light, and perhaps deepened with further experience. Sr Jarvis tells of a ward sister with whom she worked:

Sr Jarvis: ... I absorbed her sort of ... efficiency, if you like. She was efficient to the nth degree. You just couldn't catch her out at all. (Int. 10-3: 27)

Later, working with other Sisters, Sr Jarvis learns that there are other qualities which help to make a ward work well.

Sr Jarvis: [...] But up until I worked in Coronary Care Unit, I didn't realize that, yes you can be efficient, but it's also important that you enjoy your work and you make the most of the people that you're working with. (Int. 10-3: 27)

With the experience of working with several ward sisters, the Sisters recognize the possibility of different ways of practising nursing. Thus while the Sisters may trustingly and unreflectively absorb others' patterns of nursing early in their careers, only later as they gain experience, are the patterns understood and changed or adopted freely.

Learning as picking up

Learning as picking up is linked to nursing practice as an active process of coping in the situation. The Sisters pick up ways of working with patients and the ward while they are in the situation. It is perhaps the most common way of learning in everyday practice. Learning may begin with noticing, but picking up includes a movement in understanding and acting as well. It is often impossible for the Sisters to identify when and how they 'come to know', as picking up is so often gradual and seemingly incidental.

Picking up happens over time in practice. Sr Dunn tells about how she learns to respond appropriately to patients with chronic, draining chest wounds.

Sr Dunn: I think you learn to say to them 'you're looking better'. [. . .] . . . . I probably found it, just by talking to them in the right way. It was probably better than saying, 'Well, where does it hurt' or 'Is it sore there? Well we better get an X-ray, we better get the doctor to see you'. [. . .]
M.M.:   So at one point in time you did say those kinds of things.
Sr Dunn: Oh yes. I think so. I think just through dealing with them every week, and probably getting a bit fed up listening to them every week. Think 'Oh well I'll have to sort this out'. And try [. . .] and NOT make it as if they've got a disease. It's just a part of their life now. [. . .]
I think it can be wearing on you when somebody comes in and there's always something wrong. I think it would be dead easy to say, 'Oh what's it going to be this week'. [. . .] And getting the doctor. [. . .] I think probably that the patient does that, cause he's frightened as well. And if you can get them over that and try to get the message over to them that' they're not going to come to any harm because of this. And 'or we'll deal with it' and it's not very nice but it's not really that great a problem. And then you find that they're not full of complaints every week. (Int. 4-3: 22–23)

Because she is in the situation of having to 'listen to them every week', Sr Dunn begins to hear the meaning of their complaints. She comes to understand how her approach is not helpful, notices the possibility of a different approach, and changes, finding a more appropriate way, 'just by talking to them in the right way'.

The Sisters also pick up what to do from making mistakes and being caught out. The mistakes may be their own, or they may be those of others. Sr Baxter learns about the importance of clearly communicating with relatives from observing the difficulties encountered by a ward sister with whom she was working (Int. 2-1: 17–18). With mistakes, what is important to the Sisters is:

Sr Grant: . . . . not making the same mistakes twice. Knowing what your mistakes were and saying, 'Next time I don't do it that way'. [chuckle] (Int. 7-3: 39)

The Sisters monitor and change their practice because they care about their patients and their practice. They value doing their job well.

Picking up comes from being in the situation, '. . . it's learning by practising' (Int. 6-3: 33). Over time, Sr Baxter learns how to unobtrusively monitor students and staff; Sr Ellis learns to make fine discriminations in the smells of different wounds. Through experience, Sr Jarvis learns just how fast a clot can form in a bladder. Her theoretical knowledge about clot formation takes on new relevance as she learns how fast it happens, and how the resistance in the catheter during the irrigation actually feels. The Sisters 'learn in their fingertips', in their sense of timing and pacing, from being in the situation.

Learning as picking up implies a finely-tuned feedback mechanism. The Sisters are attuned: they notice what is going on; they pick up what went well, or what went wrong; they listen and hear, seeing the possibilities for alternative ways of understanding and acting. The situations and people in them matter; the Sisters willingly change their actions to become more effective practitioners.

THE ROLE OF NOTICING IN LEARNING

Noticing plays a key role in the movement of experiencing. It seems to provide for understanding and acting on the possibilities in the situation. In so doing it allows for learning.[1] As discussed in the last chapter, the Sisters become ever more skilled at noticing fine distinctions in everyday situations.

The Sisters notice the little things throughout their workday: the subtle (and not so subtle) changes to familiar patterns which trigger new thoughts or actions. They recognize what is not there and what is there that shouldn't be. They see patterns at a glance, such as when Sr Inglis glances around the ward and learns how the work is going. Over time, the Sisters continually deepen their web of understanding of patterns and sharpen their abilities to notice.

Attuned to the situations they find themselves in, the Sisters constantly notice the possibilities inherent in the situation. Sr Baxter tells about how she has come to be able to notice when patients 'haven't picked up' what the doctor has said.

Sr Baxter: There's no set teaching involved. I think it's probably ... observation. And you can perceive ... you can just feel something in some people. And some people sometimes start to say something and stop.
And you can either pick up on that. And if you do, you can maybe probe deeper into what they're thinking. I think it's basically observation. It's something that's there by looking, and listening often. By what you don't say, by what you don't see as a nurse. Often you tend to see a bit more. (Int. 2-1: 23)

Through close observation and attention, stemming from their care and concern, the Sisters pick up small changes in their patients' demeanour. They are attuned to the silence as much as to the noise. They get feedback on their actions and alter their approach, constantly monitoring the patients' responses. Through this process the Sisters learn more about the patients and their practice. Often the feedback cannot easily be put into words.

Sr Dunn: [. . .] You certainly get something between a nurse and her patients. Some kind of feeling. Well the nurse gets a feeling from a patient when she's done all she can for them. (Int. 4-3: 30)

The Sisters are constantly attuned to their patients, picking up the subtle as well as the not so subtle cues. Although they continually adjust their own actions for the patient, their concentration is on their work, not on their own performance. However, they notice the effects of their performance on the patients and on the work of the ward.

Noticing is not always at a glance. When the Sisters figuratively or literally take a step back to get another perspective on the problem, they reframe the problem, allowing different things to become salient, to stand out in the situation. In noticing differently, a new avenue for clinical judgement is opened. Although the framing of problems may be at the heart of clinical judgement (Schön 1983), noticing is central. It provides the material with which to formulate and frame the problem. The Sisters often actively help students to reframe

problems in their work. In handover reports, they often prompt noticing, 'Does that make you think?' (W3D3: 2); 'What else would you look for?' (W3D4: 17). In their own practice and in guiding others, the Sisters open new possibilities through noticing.

Keeping fresh: continuing to notice

There are times when noticing is diminished. During times of illness, or when the Sister is newly back from holiday, she is sometimes not as involved in the situation as she usually is. Sr Calder describes her feelings on her first day back at work following a relaxing holiday.

Sr Calder: And that was alien to me. Sort of sitting back and being relaxed, instead of, you know, getting on with it. Because I know I have always got to be a jump ahead to maintain this workload, and get as much as possible out ... of the little we've got. [. . .] But yesterday I was a part of that canvas. I was sitting back at one stage. [. . .] I was aware of this. I thought, 'I should be doing something, I should be doing something'. And when I got home at night I thought, 'I could have done my pharmacy'. It was all about going through what I could have been doing. But at the time, it never crossed my mind. (Int. 3-3: 17–18)

The Sisters avoid being only 'part of the canvas'. Keeping one step ahead and noticing small changes demands an active, involved stance. When they do not have that active stance, engaged in the rhythm of the work, they fail to notice.

Confidence enhances the Sisters' abilities to notice subtle changes, but the Sisters guard against the over-confidence or complacency which limits noticing. Although they take their knowledge for granted, the Sisters actively work to avoid taking patients for granted. They have different ways of keeping themselves fresh in order to notice.

Sr Ellis: You know it surprises me. You see people coming in and they're sort of unwell for a day and the next day they're up and around. When you see the children. I mean when they come back from theatre they look TERRIBLE, they're so pale and and it always amazes me when you see them in a few hours. I still always ... I have a fear of ... anaesthetics.
And when patients come back from theatre they always look terrible. It was since the first patient I ever saw when I started my training. I thought he was going to die. [. . .] And afterward I couldn't believe it

when he got well. And I still never am completely comfortable until a few hours after they recover from their anaesthetic. I don't think that's a bad thing. I think sometimes you can become too confident. [. . .] You cannot become too confident. And you try and make sure the nurses know that there are always complications. You should be aware and to watch for that. (Int. 5-1: 15–16)

Sr Ellis actively recalls her first patient who surprised her with his ability to recover from the anaesthetic. She cherishes this memory and uses it to stop herself from becoming complacent and to keep herself noticing. Like Sr Ellis, the other Sisters take something which was important, surprising or shocking at the time to serve as a touchstone in their current practice. The meaning in the original situation is retained along with a continuing, deeper meaning which they use to help them notice.

The repetition which dulls or constrains noticing is a particular problem on wards with a high turn-over of patients with similar conditions. It is also a problem for very experienced Sisters whose experience allows them to view a vast number of conditions as routine. One morning, Sr Calder notices a young person on his way out of the ward.

Sr Calder: [He] was absolutely petrified of going to theatre and I hadn't picked that up preoperatively. And he was only going for something minor. But completely uptight. And . . . . I just felt that I hadn't been with that one long enough and taken time. [. . .] I tried to reassure him on his way out the door. But you know he was on his way by that time, which I felt was too late. And I hadn't picked it up earlier. [. . .] I felt I had fallen down because I hadn't picked it up before then. (Int. 3-2: 15–19)

Whilst the turnover of patients and workflow is constant, Sr Calder expects herself to pick up on the individual patients' concerns. When she misses some, she is reminded that the repetition she is experiencing is affecting her ability to notice.

Situations like these serve to jog the Sisters' understanding of their own practice. Sr Calder consciously examines what is happening to her when she fails to notice; Sr Hanna rethinks the line of reasoning she will use when examining women who come in with pelvic inflammations; Sr Ellis consciously remembers her fright about not knowing if a patient would wake up. Others

talk about how the students keep them fresh (Grp. Int. 1: 21). But, primarily, it is the patients and the Sisters' concern for them which serve as their main prompt.

Thinking about the patient, noticing all the time and being comfortable in their own practice, allows the Sisters to monitor the effects of their practices and to continue to modify them. Unlike some of their junior nurses who are so flustered in a situation that they cannot absorb 'anything from anyone' (Int. 10-2: 4), the Sisters' stance in practice allows them to continually pick up from others. They share a deep commitment to always keep their practice open to question and to take neither their practices, nor the patients, for granted.

REFLECTING: HAVING A DIALOGUE WITH EXPERIENCE

In the movement of experience, understanding deepens and changes, in part, through reflecting. The Sisters practise thoughtfully. Whilst their perceptions and actions are fluid, and frequently intuitive, they do not 'bash on' when they are stuck (Grp. Int. 1: 28). Rather they think in the midst of action.

Schön's (1983) delineation of reflecting-in-action and reflecting-on-action is useful here. Reflecting-in-action, the Sisters get a feel for the situation, pick up on concerns or changes and alter their practice to suit. Reflection is not necessarily visual, nor in words. In the care of wounds, for example, it may be by feel or smell. The Sisters also reflect in the midst of action more deliberately and consciously as they 'take a step back' to get a new perspective on a problem, as they link and compare aspects of a current situation with previous experiences, and when they sit down to think through a discharge plan. This could be considered deliberative rather than calculative rationality.

According to Dreyfus & Dreyfus (1986), deliberative rationality is characterized by intuitively contemplating differences and experiencing a situation in light of previous situations. Approaches are planned from a consideration of the relevance and adequacy of past experiences which seem to underlie a current intuition. This is in contrast to calculative rationality which is drawing inferences from isolated, objective, abstract facts that describe the problematic situation. As they reflect-in-action, the Sisters stay within the situation, directing their attention to the patient and the ward.

In the midst of their workdays, there are few occasions for the Sisters to reflect on their practice, on their understandings of their own noticing and acting in practice. That is not to say reflecting-on-practice does not occur, but the Sisters' attention is far more frequently focused on the happenings in practice. The Sisters more commonly learn in the midst of experiencing practice than through separately reflecting on their practice.

Linking experiences

Throughout their everyday practice, the Sisters make links and connections. Reflection often starts in the form of a question which stems from noticing such a link. Sr Baxter tells of when she was a new Ward Sister, and began to notice things were not being 'done properly'. She linked this to her senior staff nurse who 'appeared so confident'.

Sr Baxter: [B]ecause I was a wee bit insecure, I had let her lead me into a false sense of security. Because I thought she knew exactly what she was doing. And I found out that she didn't. And maybe from there I started to think now, 'How can I organize my workload and organize the nurses and check on them without actually breathing down their necks all the time?' (Int. 2-3: 14)

Noticing that the staff nurse is not as competent as she appears to be opens the possibility for Sr Baxter to find a different way to monitor the nurses' work. Her questions are framed in action and pose the way for considering action differently. She begins to develop new approaches, such as finding discreet ways to accompany a nurse while she dresses a wound. In practices such as these, the Sisters make links, calling upon past experiences to reframe present understandings, in order to act differently in the future.

The Sisters are constantly comparing (cf. Clark 1991). They compare the smell of a dressing to normal wound smells; a patient's recovery to a normal recovery; the settling in process of a student to how students usually settle into a ward. They use comparisons to help students and patients learn. Sr Calder calls on a patient to recognize what his normal limb can do and to compare his progress in moving his impaired limb (W3D4: 5). She calls on students to notice the similar responses of patients to surgery on different limbs. The Sisters themselves learn through comparing.

The Sisters compare similarities and differences, both gross and subtle. They compare situation to situation and sometimes only aspects of a situation. In her second interview, Sr Baxter reviews what has been going on in the ward over the past few months. She tells about several patients who have had colostomies, yet are recovering differently. As she tells about each situation, links emerge: links of age, diagnosis, type of surgery, results of surgery, complications and how each is progressing, how their family relationships affect their recovery, how they feel about the colostomy, and what is most important in their recovery. In comparing, Sr Baxter wonders at the differences among women and their families in coping with grave illness. Her comparisons disclose the meanings in the situations for her.

Sr Baxter: The fact I suppose that you've got to be humble because Christmas was coming and Christmas is so commercialized these days and the only thing that she wanted for Christmas was the gift of life. And come Christmas Day she felt that that was what she had got. The best Christmas present she had got was the chance of having another year with her husband or however long it was, and for that she was grateful. Material things weren't of any importance. (Int. 2-2: 25)

Sometimes the meanings revealed are personal meanings for the Sisters as well. Personal links are also made between patients' situations and the Sisters' own family experiences as they consider their approach to a situation.

Sr Calder: You know I think, 'Would I like my Mum to have that? Would I like my Father to be like that?' When you see some of them, what's happening to them. Would I have liked that to happen to him? (Int. 3-3: 44–45)

Links and comparisons made by the Sisters are not unidimensional, nor simple. They are complex and temporal in nature. They open the possibility for noticing both continuity and discontinuity. Comparing and linking enables meaning to come forth.

Remembering: it comes running back to me

Linking not only occurs among aspects of current situations. As they move through their workday, the Sisters call upon their memory of a large number of details, integrating them into their understanding of patients, their recovery, and current situations in the ward. They seem to remember where each person is in the course of recovery, and link this to what they notice at the time. When Sr Calder helps Mr Ferry plan to go home, she does not specifically ask about walking with crutches on stairs, as she remembers Mr Ferry using crutches when he came into hospital (even though the memory is not in the front of her mind). The Sisters make links between what they notice throughout their workday with patients and what they already know about the patients.

Sr Fraser finishes the drug round and is in the medication room when a student comes in and tells her that Mrs Garson has vomited her supper :: Sr Fraser says, 'That's odd :: That happened when she came back [from the liver scan the previous day]'. (W6D5: 12)

The Sisters experience patients in an historical context. When they sense something different or unexpected about a person, they link the current situation to previous experiences with them. They put the present instance in the context of a norm or pattern and note possible meanings in the variance. Constantly noticing, the Sisters pick up 'bits and pieces' which they bring to bear hours and days later when assessing a comment or situation. They are continually learning about the patients and the ward.

Just as the Sisters remember details about patients throughout a day, so they remember some patients after they have gone home. There are only a few patients who 'stick in your mind' (Int. 4-2: 44), particularly on wards with a high turnover of patients. 'Routine' patients who progress normally are not memorable for the Sisters. Patients who have a difficult-to-solve nursing problem or who are particularly impressive people are remembered. So are those whom the Sister gets to know because they are in the ward repeatedly or for a much longer than usual period of time. The Sisters also remember patients who help them to learn something about themselves. This may be why so many patients in the Sisters' early months of training are remembered. With increased competence and comfort in situations, patients do not stick in the Sisters' minds so vividly. Also with increased experience, the range of normal variations broadens, making fewer patients particularly memorable (Int. 3-2: 11–13). For the most part, patients are remembered when a particular context is evoked: only a few are remembered outright.

Sometimes memories are especially vivid. Sr Dunn tells of her first death.

Sr Dunn: I think I got a shock. I can still picture that man. [. . .] He was a big man. I can still see him sat up in bed. I think you never forget that. Well I mean that was 20 odd years ago. And that's just something that sort of stays with you 'cause you've also got that wee picture there you can go back to. (Int. 4-3: 5)

Some situations like this are remembered outright and are not linked to present nursing practice. Other times, the Sister consciously links previous experiences with her current approaches. In the midst of caring for a patient, the Sister may compare her experience in this situation to her experience with previous patients. Most times, the links the Sisters make seem neither conscious nor specific.

Sr Jarvis: I don't know that I think of specific patients um . . . I don't think I thought of anyone specific when that happened to him. I didn't. I just remember having been through this before. (Int. 10-2: 27)

Such memories are often less visual but they disclose the possibilities in situations. The memory of 'being through this before' seems to evoke confidence and knowing.

The Sisters use such links and memories to assist learners. Sr Inglis helps a student faced with a complex patient to draw on her experiences of competently dealing with each aspect of the technology surrounding the patient. By breaking it down into parts, and remembering her past successful experiences, the student sees the possibility of handling a more complex patient (W9D2-1: 3–4). The Sisters help the learners to recognize that they have previous experiences which can be linked to current situations. They help the students to use their capacity to remember. Constantly drawing upon memories of previous situations and making links, the Sisters create a deep web of situational understanding.

Telling about the experience of practice

Part of reflecting in practice is telling about the experience of practising. In everyday practice, during the handover reports, throughout the work-day and outwith the work situation, the Sisters tell about their experiences with patients and the work of the ward. Telling about experiences usually happens in conversation with themselves or with others; some is in writing. It seems that telling about experience takes at least four forms. One is recapping, or reviewing for the purpose of solving problems or confirming decisions. Closely linked to this first form is a second, making sense through telling. Disparate elements are joined when telling about a patient or situation and new sense is made. In the third form, telling allows for the naming of phenomena, and in naming, the phenomena take on new importance or relevance. Lastly, telling is a form in which knowing about practice is passed on to others.

Recapping and confirming

Telling is often a form of solving problems, reviewing practices and making plans. The Sisters talk to themselves about their patients and their practices, sometimes silently, sometimes out loud.

Sr Aitkin: [W]hen I go to bed I do a little ward round in my brain. [. . .] I just go around every patient and [. . .] I think have I done anything for those people today. 'Ah tadatadadada ah Mavis I gave a placebo to. Was that the right thing to do? Well yes because she's quite happy, and . . . no problems. She'll sleep well tonight because she had her MST.[2] Glynis, well Glynis is a bit grumpy tonight maybe she'll . . . ' But I'll switch off eventually. [. . .]
M.M.: Do you ever come in with new things on your...
Sr Aitkin: Oh yes. Often when I'm walking up to work in the morning I think well I've changed my mind about that. We'll do such and such for Mrs so-and-so today. Yesterday while I was giving the report it came to my mind, because the weather was nice, to take them out for a walk. (Int. 1-1: 35)

Hearing themselves may bring out new meanings in the situation. Sr Calder is talking to me as she makes follow-up appointments for discharged patients. She is thinking aloud.

'He has an ulna and radius. He's a Thursday. Yes, he's definitely a Thursday. I've told you, so I've convinced myself.'
We then talked about it. She said, 'Talking out loud — It [what she has said] sounds right. I was wondering where does one differentiate between a hand and an arm.' [Thursday is the general fracture clinic, Wednesday is the hand clinic.] (W3D2: 7–8)

Articulating thoughts allows for a new framing or focusing of a situation, problem or solution. It reveals new meanings. In all instances, telling about experiences places those experiences in language. And through language, the meanings in the experiences are disclosed (Taylor 1985). As the Sisters tell about their practices, they preserve and extend those practices by focusing them (Dreyfus 1987).

Making sense

Telling about experience may prompt new connections. In telling me about what they are doing, the Sisters often say, as Sr Inglis does, 'I don't think I've consciously thought of that before' (Int. 9-3: 28). Bringing hidden practices into conversation enables new meaning to come forward. Here Sr Grant tells about similarities between two patients and discusses their families.

Sr Grant: I think we got to know them very well. We understood their strengths and their weaknesses. And [we] liked them on a personal level; found them admirable. Not always easy but . . . the relationships were very satisfying.
I've never thought about that link, you know. I think it's very true, the link's stronger between the relatives than it is between the two patients. (Int. 7-2: 13)

The link was there, but hadn't popped into her mind. Making new links creates a new sense of connectedness; new meanings are found in experiences. Telling about experiences may not overtly change the Sisters' own practices, but it may change their understanding and how they notice. Telling can be described as a process of noticing which opens the potential for learning.

Naming practice and experience

Naming practices can bring new awareness. Sr Fraser tells about learning the meaning of 'gently mobilizing' in her first ward as a student working with a staff nurse and a particular patient.

Sr Fraser: In the morning she was raised on one pillow for her breakfast with her towel by her side. And she was bed bathed, and it was a full bed bath. And she got up to go to the toilet and we made her bed and she sat in the chair by the bed. And then she was actually put back to bed afterwards. And then she got up again in the afternoon to sit and go through. (Int. 6-3: 13)

Naming the timing and pacing experienced with the patient and staff nurse as 'the way you "gently mobilized"'allows Sr Fraser to understand an experience as something. Naming an experience or practice can also provide the Sister with a means for pointing out hitherto tacit aspects of her practice to students. Naming is different than affixing a label, as Griffin (1988) writes: 'An experience that is named in one way at one time can well be understood differently later and the interpretation reconstructed as the person grows and develops'.

Naming enables recognition and interpretation. It reveals meaning. Naming a process is also empowering (Griffin 1987). It puts the experience into a public space, articulating it and bringing it into focus.

Sharing experience

Telling about experiences enables the Sisters to share their understanding and their practice.

M.M.: What's the most useful way of talking about your experience? [. . .]
Sr Ellis: Well mainly with sort of colleagues on the ward. And even when you go down to tea and you speak to . . . But mainly people within the unit, really, [and] the post basic nurses [. . .] For example Mrs Sampson's [facial rebuilding] operation. There are not a lot of these operations done. And so we're able to say, 'Well there's not a lot done but what we've experienced is this, this and this. And we had this lady and how we feel . . . That they all look the same, these people, you know, men or women; these people that have an ear removed and a facial palsy. And they all seem to look the same, the same face, with no facial expression'. [. . .] Before they're all individuals and

afterwards they all seem to look . . . And that's something to be prepared for or to be aware of. (Int. 5-3: 32)

In handover reports the Sisters place observations such as amounts of drainage, vital signs and distances walked in the context of the person and the course of recovery: 'We colour it in' (W8D4: 8). The Sisters often tell how they were able to accomplish a task with a patient or achieve something in the system. For example, Sr Fraser tells an oncoming nurse about the process which she used to get hold of the Resident when the telephone system was down (W6D5: 8). As much as they are exchanges of information, the report times are times of sharing experiences. They are important for the Sisters.

Sr Ellis: But I think it's a fact that so much can be taught to people through theory but, you know it's essential to have some training, some background, some knowledge. But I think really at the end of the day the experience that you've gained and . . . looking at your experience, and discussing it with others and using it in a positive way, is the most important thing, I think, the overall most important thing. (Int. 5-3: 31)

Talking about experiences allows the Sisters to explore their feelings about patients and situations. It provides an opportunity for the Sisters to find new meanings in experiences and to come to terms with difficult situations. In their everyday work of encountering death and dealing with the intimate '. . . most private aspects of people's lives . . .' (Fagin & Diers 1984), this is necessary. '[W]e need to go through it . . . [. . .] and we see it and we try and talk' (Int. 5-3: 34).

Telling about experiences enables the Sisters to learn in and from their experiences. Sharing experiences is a 'powerful way of clarifying confusion, identifying appropriate questions and reaching significant insights' (Knights 1985). In telling, the links and connections which the Sisters make between their present situation and remembered situations are revealed. When they tell about their experiences in practice, the Sisters are not detached, rather they remain engaged, concerned about what is going on. Often telling about practice brings with it a hint of the journey towards greater understanding of themselves and their nursing practice.

LEARNING WITH OTHER PEOPLE

Nursing is practice with people and the Sisters continuously learn from the people around them. Patients figure centrally. The Sisters talk of ward sisters, staff nurses, doctors and family and friends as being influential. Perhaps understandably, these experienced Sisters mention a teacher only once. Three aspects of learning with people stand out in the Sisters' accounts. The first is learning about ways of being a nurse and a person simply by being with patients and other nurses. The second relates to the importance of being challenged and given responsibility yet being supported at the same time. The third concerns the inter-connection of the Sisters' practice and their lives 'outside'.

Learning by being with others

Each of the Sisters tells about people they had worked with over the course of their careers who made a strong impression on them as nurses. Sr Grant tells what makes certain people influential:

Sr Grant: .... I think the thing they have in common is that they all have attributes that I would like to have myself. I admire them and would like to behave as they do. So in that experience . . . In that way I've modelled myself on them. Although I think they were probably quite different sorts of people with different styles. They all had things that I particularly valued.
M.M.: Mm hmm. Have these people come along or been with you at particularly influential times in your life?
Sr Grant: Um .... well because they were there it became influential. (Int. 7-3: 35)

The Sisters describe learning from how their own ward sisters practised nursing: how they ran their wards, talked to patients, worked with the medical staff, coped with stress or created a caring atmosphere in which to work.

Sr Jarvis: I know that she taught me an awful lot. She was from an intensive care background. And at this time I had never set foot in an intensive care unit in my training apart from head injuries which I'd hated. She showed me that the confidence and knowledge that she had gained doing intensive care and the intensive care course had helped her in a general ward situation.

And it had also given her confidence in dealing with medical staff. She wasn't prepared to just say, 'They're the medical staff, they know best', and would leave it at that. She realized that the patient was the most important person. And she did whatever she could do to make sure that that patient was looked after properly. And if that meant going over the head of whoever was looking after them at the time then she would do it.

Her style was very different to what mine is now. I know that. But those sorts of things that she taught me I've never forgotten. (Int. 10-3: 24–25)

The Sisters not only learned about concrete aspects of nursing practice, they learned different ways of being nurses.

Being challenged and supported

Sometimes the Sisters were challenged to think about nursing in a different way.

Sr Grant: [It was] at a time when I felt very disillusioned about nursing and was ready to call it a day. And I went to [the teacher] and said, 'This is not for me, I'm going to call it a day'. And she basically said to me in a quite sympathetic way, 'Don't you dare opt out — After all the effort I've made?'. [. . .] And, 'If you're not happy with it, you change it. You do not leave'. And in a very nice way. I came back and I realized what she'd said. 'And how are you going to change it?' (Int. 7-3: 36–37)

The Sisters described influential nurses and doctors as being supportive.

Sr Grant: Well I think perhaps the only person I can really remember being supportive in that situation was our senior Registrar [. . .] Who himself was very organized and a good administrator, an interested administrator. . . . . . . We consulted one another. He always seemed to know what was going on. And I think between us, we worked out what our different roles would be. (Int. 7-3: 8)

Being supported includes being respected and being helped to find ways in which to handle the responsibilities of the position. Most of the Sisters tell about feeling supported and challenged as a senior student or in their first staff job. Being supported includes being challenged with responsibility, but having enough help to successfully handle it. Sr Calder tells about her experience as a young staff nurse with a ward sister who was considered to be an 'ogre'.

Sr Calder: Sisters were always around in those days. And she would come up and say to me, 'Do you know anything about diabetics? What do you know about your insulin and all this jazz?' I said 'Oh, what do you want to know?' And you know, 'Well do you know where it comes from and Islets of Langerhans da da da'. I can't remember all the specifics. 'Oh' I said, 'No'. You know by this time, we did communicate and I mean she appreciated me and I appreciated her. 'Right then.' So she would rattle off something to me. And I thought 'OK', standing up. And then we would have a diabetic [lesson at the handover report] 'Tell me.' She'd come to the first year nurse. And she'd ask [the students] a question about diabetes. And they wouldn't know. 'Staff Nurse would you tell them?' And I would tell them. And she'd only told me 5 minutes before.

[...] She made sure that I knew before she ever did that. But she did it. And then it made the staff nurse look better in the students' eyes. And I mean, I knew quite a bit of it but sometimes there were bits that I didn't know. But she had checked it all out that I did know. (Int. 3-3: 36)

Ward sisters and staff nurses who were supportive 'inspired great confidence' (Int. 7-3: 37). They 'gave [the Sister] the courage' to try (Int. 6-3: 36). They believed in the Sisters' abilities to nurse, and to nurse well. Their standards were good, they knew their specialty and they 'ran' a good ward.

Ward sisters who refused to let the Sisters take on responsibility and who blocked involvement in care, stymied growth.

Sr Ellis: [The ward sister] knew all about [the specialty of surgical procedures], but she never shared that information. You ASSISTED her. She did the pre-med, she did the dressings, she did the doctors' rounds, and even as a staff nurse you assisted her with everything. And she'd be here from 7 o'clock in the morning until midnight every day if she could. And so really in the end we were learning very little. And in her absence we were keeping the place going, really. You weren't making any decisions or changing anything. You were just keeping the place ticking over until she came back. We were frightened to let anyone go home in case it was wrong.

So, after I became a staff nurse and she'd retired I really sort of felt as if ... Although I knew how to run a ward basically, I didn't really know anything particular about the specialty apart from what I'd read in a book, or someone else had told me. So I think I felt as if I started from scratch and I've just learned from experience. (Int. 5-1: 19)

Supportive ward sisters set up situations to help nurses become confident and see new possibilities.

Sr Jarvis: [...] I can remember [Sister] sitting down and chatting with me about what I was going to plan on doing, and conveying to me the sort of experience that she had gained from intensive care. And how she thought it could enhance what I was doing. (Int. 10-3: 25)

All of the Sisters have worked with ward sisters who have recognized their potential and have challenged and supported them to realize possibilities the Sisters themselves have not yet seen. These ward sisters have shared themselves and their experiences with the Sisters.

Living and learning

All of the Sisters have ways 'not to take work home', but they recognize the intertwining of their experience in nursing practice with their whole life experience. Families and friends strongly influence the Sisters' learning. Like Sr Aitkin's flatmate who helped her to see her practices from a different perspective (Int. 1-1: 29) and Sr Baxter's granny who taught her to get along with people (Int. 2-3: 12). Friends and family members help the Sisters come to new understandings. What they learn in their life outside nursing impacts on their practice.

Sr Inglis: I certainly feel that bringing up two teenagers, I'd like to think makes me a bit closer to these youngsters [student nurses]. [...] You know I see both sides of it. They're young, they've got all these stresses in life, but nevertheless they've chosen nursing to come in to. It's a disciplined profession. So they jolly well have to work hard. [...] Yes. I think it gives you a good insight into how they tick. (Int. 9-3: 23–24)

Also, what the Sisters learn in practice impacts on their outside lives:

Sr Inglis: .... You see my husband would say I've become a much tougher person, harder. And I think I probably have.
M.M.: In what way?
Sr Inglis: I think I probably would have given in an awful lot in our early marriage. And he would have always won the day. Now that might have come anyway, whether I had been a nurse or not. I think that might just have been experience doing that. But I can certainly stand my ground now. And I do it with doctors, with the hierarchy. And with visitors, if I have to. And with patients if I really have to. [...] And if a decision has to be made in the ward and it doesn't suit everyone, then that's too bad if it's the decision that I have really thought about. Because there's no way you're going to please everybody. (Int. 9-3: 24)

What the Sisters gain from people outwith nursing affects them, and therefore has the potential to affect their practice. Conversely, what the Sisters learn in practice affects them as people. This is particularly so in the case of learning from patients.

There has been little direct mention of how patients figure into learning yet they are the main source of the Sisters' experience and are thus the primary teachers. Learning about the meaning of illness, and the character of people they care for, are among the sources of greatest satisfaction for the Sisters. 'She [the patient] gives a lot back to us, so I think you can learn a lot from how she's coping and her spirit' (Int. 6-2: 22). Knowing how patients help them to learn, the Sisters actively encourage learner nurses to find out how illness affects patients and how they can most help.

[Sr Aitkin] advises the student to 'Talk to her about her symptoms . . . You can read it in books, but talking with patients is the way you learn it'. (W1D1: 4)

Being attuned to patients and their concerns enables the Sisters to gain from their patients in understanding and in satisfaction. The Sisters learn not only from their own experiences, they also learn from the experiences of patients and colleagues. Learning with others is part of experiencing nursing.

CONCLUDING COMMENTS

For the Sisters, experience in everyday practice is the foremost source of understanding how to care for patients and how to run their wards. In everyday practice, they learn, whether or not they intend to. Learning is part and parcel of experiencing nursing practice. Noticing plays a special role in relation to experiencing. It produces an opening of possibility which allows for the movement in experience. Into this gap comes learning which gives the movement its direction and influences the quality and quantity of change. Learning is much like the wind. It is impossible to grasp but its presence and influence are unmistakable.

Experiencing takes many forms, but characteristic of all experiences is the Sisters' involvement which allows them to grasp the meanings inherent in their practice and experiences with patients and others. Constant noticing, coupled with memory and making linkages, enable the Sisters to come to 'realize', to understand. Coming to realize is like the hermeneutic circle, where parts are identified and understood, then the whole is grasped, causing different sense to be made of the parts.

In their practice, the Sisters are continually open to new experience. Their conversations are dialogues in which they listen and come to new understandings of what they hear and experience. Their actions work in much the same way, with their bodies becoming more skilled as they move through practice.

The Sisters' learning is much like a journey, one in which their openness to experience helps them along the way. The journey leads them to become experienced in practice, and to a greater understanding of themselves as nurses and people. It is easier to track the Sisters' journey when they are newly in a situation: unfamiliar situations and new experiences lead to conscious reflection which is easy to grasp. It is harder to track subtle differences in a person whose experience and situational understanding is already complex.

It is difficult to say if the form of experience and learning has changed over the years among the Sisters. Certainly the focus of their experiences changes as time goes on. It seems likely that they have always been aware of what is going on in a ward and they have always noticed particularly. A clue to this comes from their awareness of the different facets of the characters of the ward sisters with whom they worked earlier in their careers. None of the people described by the Sisters as influential are 'cardboard' characters. The Sisters describe their current experiences with the same attention to salient details. Although they recognize themselves in less experienced nurses, they are no longer at this point. Their confidence and ability to handle situations have moved them beyond the others. What opens up through noticing and where they look for solutions to problems are different. They also continually seek new information. They seek the hearing of others that dialogue can bring. Their confidence removes the threat from many things which may once have been threatening. They enjoy their experiences and their journey.

This book has also been something of a journey as we have explored the terrain of the Sisters' experiences and their practice, and investigated the flow of their practising and experiencing. It remains now to complete this journey and to see what it tells us about the nature of everyday experience in nursing practice.

Notes

[1] See also Boud & Walker (1990) who characterize noticing as 'an act of becoming aware' (p 68), an activity that plays an important role in reflection and in learning from experience.

[2] Long-acting morphine.

8

Summary, conclusions and beyond

INTRODUCTION

So far in this book, the everyday experience in nursing practice of 'experienced' surgical ward sisters has been uncovered and explored. In this chapter, I shall recapitulate on the major themes which have been developed throughout the book and draw out some of their implications. Before moving on to that discussion, it may be useful to recall the origins of this research.

The original aim of the research was to explore the nature of everyday experience in nursing practice with a view to gaining an understanding of how that everyday experience contributes to the development of nursing expertise. I came to this research from the position of an educational administrator in nursing who, like others in my position, made administrative decisions and planned academic courses based on the common-sense understanding that nurses learned through their everyday experience in practice. Indeed, this commonsense understanding is such that the need for a certain number of months or years of 'related clinical experience' is written into job descriptions and continuing education course admission requirements. Without the necessary experience, nurses are neither hired, nor admitted to courses.

However, everyday experience, possibly because it is so familiar, is usually taken for granted: it has not been the subject of systematic investigation. Perhaps it is not surprising then, that such experience is often accorded less worth than academic preparation as a source of knowledge and skills. This is particularly so in North America. Thus, with the understanding that nurses in the United

Kingdom have a reputation for providing good, clinical, bedside care, and that pragmatic, practical experience is strongly valued, I chose to undertake this study among Scottish nurses.

It will be recalled that I originally sought to study nurses who were considered to be 'expert' surgical nurses. I found, however, that there were difficulties with using the term, 'expert': it was said to be 'too American' and seldom, if ever, used to describe nurses in direct clinical practice. Instead, the two Directors of Nursing Service agreed to identify 'excellent, experienced' surgical nurses. They identified with ease 10 nurses who met the criteria first used by Benner (1984) to identify expert nurses. Significantly, eight of the nurses were ward sisters; the other two fulfilled part of a ward sister role. Locating experience and excellence in clinical practice at this position is not unusual in the National Health Service. The ward sister is generally thought to be the 'repository of clinical expertise' (Lathlean 1987 p 16). This selection of ward sisters also may reflect the lack of specialist, clinical positions in Scottish hospitals, as well as the relative lack of full-time, experienced staff nurses in the 'general' surgical wards at the time of the study. Although the clinical grading structure has the potential to create alternative routes for clinical advancement, at the time the nurses were selected, Rogers and Powell's contention held true: the existing career structure in the NHS '... does not enable a nurse to retain a major clinical involvement or responsibility beyond the grade of a Sister' (Rogers & Powell 1983).

With the selection of ward sisters as the experienced, excellent clinical nurses, an unavoidable question is raised: why is clinical practice invisible in the ward sister literature? As was seen in Chapter 3, the teaching and management aspects of the ward sister's role have been repeatedly studied, but the clinical role has been overlooked and the ward sister's clinical practice taken for granted. I would like to suggest that the clinical expertise of the ward sister, while it may be acknowledged, is undervalued. This undervaluing, I will presently argue, is linked to the nature of knowing in everyday practice which remains, for the most part, hidden from

view. Nurses in the United Kingdom are not alone in undervaluing everyday experience and knowing. I would suggest that everyday clinical practice and experience are taken for granted as readily in Canada and the United States as they are in Scotland.

Before moving to a discussion of the Ward Sisters' practices and the nature of their everyday experience, it may be opportune to recall the approach taken to the study, and why I found this to be a useful way to examine everyday, taken-for-granted experience.

Study approach

In determining an approach to the study of a phenomenon, the decision is ultimately a philosophical one. Most of the studies which have considered nursing practice and learning in experience have been in the philosophical tradition of Descartes and Husserl. In this tradition, the fundamental human situation is of a subject in a world of objects. An understanding of experience results from directing the mind towards that world or towards itself, towards its mental contents. In order to do this, Husserl suggests that we 'bracket' our everyday understanding. What this tradition overlooks, as Heidegger so aptly pointed out, is the everyday skilful coping in taken-for-granted experience. To use one of his examples: we are not aware of turning the doorknob, we are only aware of the doorknob when it sticks. When the doorknob sticks we attempt to un-stick it, and it is only when that does not work that we may need to think about the specific properties of the doorknob itself. This is the point at which Husserl begins, the point of contemplation.

Heidegger argues that what needs study before the problem of knowing, is everyday being-in-the world, as 'much if not most characteristic human activity is not guided by conscious choices, and not accompanied by aware states of mind' (Magee 1987 p 260). It would follow then that much of everyday experience in nursing practice is overlooked and taken for granted because it is skilful coping in the midst of an ongoing situation.

Unless a problem develops or a doorknob sticks, we remain unaware of the skills and knowledge essential to this coping. Thus, an approach following in the tradition of Heidegger may be a more fruitful way of examining everyday, taken-for-granted nursing experience.

In Chapters 2 and 3, I proposed that studies using hermeneutic phenomenology (e.g. Gray-Snelgrove 1982, Diekelmann 1993, Benner 1984, 1994), seemed to be the most successful in capturing the complex, situational and relational nature of experience and nursing practice. Hermeneutic phenomenology, in focusing on the person in the world, dissolves the subject-object dichotomy and enables the background meanings in shared practices and language to become visible. Therefore, through the perspective of hermeneutic phenomenology, I examined the nature and meanings of the Sisters' everyday experience in nursing practice.

A problem which I have not altogether avoided in this study is the risk of overlooking the structural interdependence of the person and society (Giddens 1982). Focusing the analysis on the inter-subjective nature of the experiences of and the relationship between the Sisters and their everyday situation has partially, but not wholly, counteracted this potential for isolating the Sisters in relation to the institution and society. If the goal of this study was explanation, an explicit connection with the broader social structures would be critical. However, as this study seeks to understand the nature of everyday experience and what it means to learn and to be 'experienced', an explicit connection is of lesser importance. The Sisters' language and practices reveal the broader social world; special attention to this aspect must await another analysis.

In order to study everyday, moment-by-moment experience in nursing practice, I interviewed the Ward Sisters about memorable and everyday experiences and observed them in ongoing practice on the ward. The study was productive of many insights about their nursing practice as well as about the nature of their everyday experience. It certainly would be possible to focus exclusively upon the nature of ward sister practice; it would

also be possible to distinguish domains of practice and competencies, as Benner (1984) and others have done. From a Canadian perspective on both British and American nursing practice, it would also be possible to examine in depth, the differences in practice which are often overlooked because the language, on the surface, is the same. I examined all of these areas on this journey, but for the purposes of this book, the core of the study is understanding the nature of taken-for-granted, moment-by-moment experience, and how it contributes to the development of expertise amongst 'experienced' ward sisters. Having said that, however, the nature and context of that practice is crucial to the argument because experience happens only in the midst of ongoing practice.

Although nursing practice could easily become the foreground, for the purposes of this book, it must remain in the background. However, it cannot be overlooked or diminished. So before moving on to the discussion of experience, the core of this book, I will briefly review what the study revealed about the nature of the Ward Sisters' nursing practice.

BEING A SURGICAL WARD SISTER

When the Sisters' practice is viewed from the vantage point of everyday experience, it is revealed to be purposeful, caring, complex, multi-faceted and patient-centred. In Chapter 5, I have described how the Sisters make the ward work in order to help individual patients towards recovery. As the section on 'Helping patients towards recovery' illustrates, the Sisters experience each patient within the temporal framework of their stay on the ward. As the Sisters organize or provide care directly to individual patients, their practices reflect an understanding of the patients' experiences in the past, how they are in the present and what possibilities there may be for the future. The Sisters become adept at picking up on subtle variations in people's responses to recovery. They also become adept at creating complex goals for seemingly innocuous activities, such as eating or bathing, which actively assist the patient towards recovery. It is this complexity yet subtlety of goals and interventions which are not adequately recognized. They do not receive the prominence they deserve in much of the current research literature on recovery from surgery (cf. Wilson-Barnett & Fordham 1982, Devine 1992).

The Sisters orchestrate the care of patients by a largely junior and transient workforce. This is characterized in Chapter 5 as 'Making the ward work'. A phrase commonly heard amongst them, 'Today's another day', expresses the temporality of their experience. The Sisters make the ward work, for the most part, on a shift-by-shift basis. The juxtaposition of their experiences of the patients individually over time in the midst of the day-by-day experience of the work of the ward is a source of creative tension. Their everyday practices reveal how this tension is played out. Their practices, which are replete with complex goals, much like Dewey's (1925) ends-in-view, are directed individually, yet are within the context of ensuring care for all the patients on the ward.

The Sisters' experiences and practices are revealed to be interlinked: they are contextual and relational. They are formed in and for the particular situations in which the Sisters find themselves. A number of examples in Chapters 4 and 5 illustrate, for instance, how the Sisters change their conversational approach to suit a particular patient, finely adjust their movements in response to the demands of a patient's wound, or intervene with finesse when a junior medical or nursing staff member is running into difficulty. Upon close examination of the interview transcripts and field notes, a process of noticing, understanding and acting was found to characterize this relational and contextual nature of the Sisters' practices. This process, a key finding of the study, was also found to be the process of experiencing practice. It will be further discussed in relation to the nature of experience.

Although nursing practice provides the ground for the main thrust of this book, a few comments may be made about the view of practice revealed by this study. In the nursing practice literature, this study sits closely to Benner's work and to the

ward sister studies. Thus it is to that work that we now turn.

This study found a somewhat different pattern of practices in comparison to Benner's competencies. Although at least seven 'domains of nursing practice' (Benner 1984) could be discerned from the analysis of the Sisters' practices, the analysis did not proceed along the line of identifying competencies, roles and domains of practice. Instead, the Sisters' practices were better understood in relation to their experience of the stay of the patient and the day-to-day working of the ward. In addition, many of the Sisters' practices address more than one role or competency. For example, when the Sisters place a patient's bed in a particular position in the ward, they do it to meet the patient's individual needs, while at the same time seeking to effect a smooth delivery of care to all the patients using the workforce at hand. The approach of domains and competencies usefully illuminates the complexity of nursing practice, but I would argue that a taxonomic form cannot adequately capture the flow of everyday experience in nursing practice.

It was argued in Chapter 3 that many studies in the ward sister literature hold that the ward sister role is a complex one, yet individual studies focus on only one part of the role. Perhaps the most influential of the studies is Pembrey's (1980), in which she describes the role of the ward sister in the management of nursing on an individualized patient basis. That role, she contends, consists of implementing the four stages of the management cycle in relation to each patient and each nurse. This study has shown that the Sisters' practices together form a complex whole which is centred on the patient. Rather than being a separate endeavour, the Sisters' management practices have been seen to be virtually inseparable from their practices concerned with helping patients towards recovery. Their practices concerned with helping junior nursing and medical staff to learn are similarly interlinked. This interlinking would seem to have important consequences for the development of the ward sister role and the education of ward sisters (charge nurses or nurse managers).

Whilst the ward sister role may need to be enhanced from a management perspective (Lathlean 1988), or for the purposes of ensuring adequate clinical education of students (UKCC 1986, NBS 1989), the findings of this study indicate that the management and education components of the role should be strengthened only within a context of caring for patients. This study has shown the need to recognize anew the value of the expertise of experienced ward sisters. Their role in assuring the quality of care for patients and learning for students is crucial. The ward sisters manage the work of the ward, ensure the quality of care and help junior staff and doctors to learn, whilst keeping the patients at the hub of all their endeavours.

Chapter 5, in particular, detailed how the Sisters practise in the midst of organizational constraints. Such everyday organizational experiences include frequently being a safety net for a transient and junior workforce; difficulties in meeting the standard of care which patients 'deserve' within a complex hospital organization with often inadequate staffing; and having authority within the ward, but not perceiving themselves to have authority within the organization. These organizational constraints echo the 'extreme work overload, staff shortages, a preponderance of inexperienced nurses, and high staff turnover', found to be barriers to expert clinical practice in the AMICAE study in California (Benner & Wrubel 1982) and reinforced by Gruber & Benner (1989). Yet in the present study, 'excellent, experienced' Scottish ward sisters were found to be practising expertly, keeping the patient at the centre of their care and helping junior staff and doctors to learn. Although they were concerned about the quality of care, they were not too busy for caring.

Although relevant findings with which to specifically link this study to the North American context are lacking, I would suggest that the physical environment and the authority of the ward sister may be two important factors to consider in comparing nursing practice between the United Kingdom and North America. In the study hospitals, the open architecture enables the Ward Sisters to monitor and attend to the patients, and supervise students in different ways than may be possible in wards where the nurse has to enter individual rooms before being able to see or communicate with the patient.

The clinical authority of the ward sister was one of the most puzzling aspects to me, as a Canadian, of understanding her practice. There seems to be a marked difference in the location and exercise of authority between the North American system of nursing as reported in the literature and the system within which the Ward Sisters work. The Sisters seem to have more authority, possibly because of their historically derived position as head of the ward. This is bolstered by their clinical knowledge and expertise. Perhaps reflecting the differences in the societies, nurses in the North American system lack that entrenched, positional authority. American nurses, particularly primary nurses, operate more from personal authority: from their clinical knowledge and knowledge of the patient (Prescott et al 1987). There are marked differences between the amount and nature of interaction between doctors and nurses reported in the US literature (Schilder 1986, Katzman & Roberts 1988) and the more frequent interaction which I observed amongst the Ward Sisters and the residents, registrars and consultants. Differences such as these would be worthwhile exploring should the opportunity present itself to compare in a comprehensive way this study's material to Benner's (1984) domains and competencies.

The discussion thus far has revealed some of the complexity of the Ward Sisters' day-by-day nursing practice. I have suggested that their everyday practices are inseparable from their experience of practice. Indeed, I would suggest that for these 'excellent, experienced' Ward Sisters, being a surgical ward sister can be characterized as being attuned to experience: the experience of patients, the experience of those with whom they work and their own experience. Being attuned to experience also appears to be the way in which the Sisters develop expertise through moment-by-moment, day-by-day practice. It is to experience and experiencing practice that we now turn.

THE NATURE OF EVERYDAY EXPERIENCE

When experience is referred to in the research literature, for example the literature on learning in experience, it is usually taken to be a non-problematic, static, spatial entity. Experience is considered to be something which a person has and can give meaning to, something that can be reflected upon retrospectively. Even in the phenomenological studies, with few exceptions (e.g. Gray-Snelgrove 1982), experience is treated as if it is non-problematic, to be examined only for the meaning it contains (the meanings in lived experience). When the focus of the studies is on everyday practices (e.g. Benner 1984, Benner et al 1992), the meanings in the experience are revealed as being relational and contextual. However, the nature of experience itself is not usually considered to be problematic, and has not been the focus of attention.

In this study, the focus of attention is directly on the nature of experiencing everyday practice. In the field notes and interviews, the Sisters' ongoing moment-by-moment experiencing, as well as their retrospective experiences, were recorded. When these field notes and interviews were examined, experience was not found to be as static nor as simple as it is usually made out to be. It was revealed to be fluid and complex, closely linked to moment-by-moment nursing practice and already imbued with meaning.

Time plays an important part in ongoing experiencing. By looking at moment-by-moment nursing practices and by examining the links among past experiences and projections for future practices, experience is found to be always in a state of flux. It becomes evident that previous experience is linked to experiencing in the present, which in turn is geared towards possibilities in the future.

The Sisters' experience was found to take many forms, ranging from intensive, vivid and memorable 'watershed' experiences, through the less emotional 'resonant' experiences of their accounts, to the most prevalent, taken-for-granted experience which accompanies most 'usual', everyday practice. Sometimes they could identify 'an experience' and tell about it as such, but more frequently experiencing was vague and elusive, and expressed by the Sisters as 'just experience'. Sometimes, experiences were immediately meaningful; what was expected was not found and the Sisters' understanding of a situation was disconfirmed. More frequently, however, the experiences were subtle, with meanings gradually unfolding over time. These more subtle, unnoticed experiences often served to extend, enrich and confirm understanding. Sometimes, after a period of time and experience, the Sister would notice a change in her understanding and 'suddenly realize'. Also, as the Sisters gained experience, different meanings in previous experiences would often emerge. Experience is not static in the past: experiencing comes from the past, is in the present and is geared towards the possibilities of the future.

This variety and complexity of experience is notable on at least two counts. In studying nursing practice from the vantage point of experience, it would seem to be important to take into account the nature of experience and the view of practice afforded by different types of experience. For example, the emotion which is evoked by many of the examples in Benner & Wrubel's important book may stem, in part, from the paradigm cases which provide the basis for much of the discussion. These paradigm cases are themselves infused with emotion: they are significant, watershed experiences for the nurses involved. The impression of nursing practice thus portrayed, while important, is somewhat skewed as it gives insufficient attention to the nursing practice which lies outwith 'paradigm' experiences. Within the context of the present study, by contrast, the meanings of the Sisters' current practices cannot be adequately understood unless the various forms of that experience are appropriately recognized. This is highlighted by the fact that as they become more experienced, the Sisters have fewer watershed experiences. At the same time, their practice does not remain static: it continues to develop and change.

Taking the complexity of experience into account is important too, when considering how learning accompanies experience. For the Sisters, becoming experienced surgical nurses seems to be a complex process, linked to their moment-by-moment practising. They seem to be learning all the time. Just as experience appears to be fluid and elusive, so too does learning in everyday practice. Learning does not seem to be as discrete a phenomenon as various experiential learning models (e.g. Kolb 1984, Boud et al 1985) would suggest. Instead, learning could be said to accompany experiencing in everyday practice and as well, to be an outgrowth of experience. Being attuned to experience is the process through which the Sisters develop expertise.

BEING ATTUNED TO EXPERIENCE

The continuous interplay between practice and experience which emerges from the Sisters' accounts and observations of their practice is explored in earlier chapters. I wish to suggest that for the 'excellent, experienced' Ward Sisters in the study, being attuned to experience is at the centre of their everyday experience in practice. Being attuned to experience carries with it a sense of openness to experience, a dialogue with others and with oneself and an understanding of knowing which goes beyond theoretical knowledge. Gadamer puts it well:

The nature of experience is conceived in terms of that which goes beyond it; for experience itself can never be science. It is in absolute antithesis to knowledge and to that kind of instruction that follows from general theoretical or technical knowledge. The truth of experience always contains an orientation towards new experience. That is why a person who is called 'experienced' has become such not only through experiences, but is also open to new experiences . . . [T]he experienced person proves to be . . . someone who is radically undogmatic; who, because of the many experiences he has had and the knowledge he has drawn from them is particularly well equipped to have new experiences and to learn from them. The dialectic of experience has its own fulfilment not in definitive knowledge, but in that openness to experience that is encouraged by experience itself. (Gadamer 1975 p 319)

Like Gadamer's 'radically undogmatic' person, the Sisters are continually open to new experience. They are open to their own experience, the experience of the medical, nursing and other staff on the wards, and most importantly perhaps, to the experience of the patients. In Chapter 7, that openness and its effect on the Sisters' learning are detailed. It is suggested that the Sisters continually keep their own practices and understanding in question, and develop ways to prevent themselves from becoming complacent and deaf to their experience.

Constantly noticing, the Sisters continually test and revise their understanding of the patient, the nursing care and the situation. Being attuned is a reflexive, comparative and connective process, through which the Sisters continually expand their capacity to notice, understand and act. The Sisters develop expertise in practice by being attuned to experience: it is the way in which they become 'experienced'. At the same time, I would argue that, for the Sisters, being attuned to experience is the ongoing process of practising nursing. This process, I would suggest, can be characterized as noticing, understanding and acting.

Noticing, understanding and acting

The process of noticing, understanding and acting, because it is the process of practising, of ongoing experiencing, is usually transparent to us. The constituents of the process cannot be readily separated and analysed. Noticing, understanding and acting are inextricably intertwined in everyday practising. Being in a particular situation, the Sister notices salient aspects of that situation, understands what they mean and acts. For instance, mid-morning she may glance around the ward, notice how the patients are faring and how the nurses are progressing with their work. Depending upon what she sees, she may smile and acknowledge the progress, help a nurse reset her priorities, help a patient back to bed, or any number of other actions which make the ward work in such a way that patients can be helped towards recovery. The Sister's understanding comes primarily from experience in previous, similar situations: it makes noticing possible. In turn, noticing and understanding are made possible because the Sister is acting: she is already in a particular situation. Finally, noticing, understanding and acting are all made possible in the first instance by the Sisters' involvement, commitment and care. Chapter 6 details this process and its links to expertise.

There is a qualitative dimension to this process. Just as the Sisters notice in the situation, they can also fail to notice. It seems that fatigue, a certain lack of involvement, or failing to understand meaning in the situation all inhibit noticing. Noticing seems to be enhanced when the Sister is confident in her own practice and it becomes transparent to her; she can broaden her focus of attention. No longer self-conscious about her own performance, the Sister can attend to the effects of nursing actions on the patients or ward situations. Noticing is also enhanced through a deep understanding of possible meanings inherent in particular situations.

Understanding is informed by both practical know-how and theoretical knowledge. It is understanding in and of a context. Although many meanings are inherent in any situation, the Sisters understand some aspects of the situation to be more salient than others. As the Sisters gain understanding of a situation, they are able to tune in on the more important aspects of similar situations. A failure to understand, or to misunderstand the meanings in a situation is also possible. The Sisters' reputations as excellent practitioners attest to the reliability of their understanding.

Like noticing and understanding, there is a qualitative aspect to acting. The Sisters' timing, pacing and suiting of their actions to particular situations derive from what they understand and how they notice. Their actions can be appropriate or inappropriate in the circumstances. Confidence seems to be a factor, both in their ability to act in certain circumstances, as well as in affecting how sure and fluid their actions are. The process of noticing, understanding and acting is a holistic one; the inseparability of body and mind is readily apparent. The Sisters' comportment, their tone of voice and their touch all play a part in experiencing and practising.

The Sisters are noticing, understanding and acting all the time in practice. It is not just the big things in practice which are included. Indeed, it is in the little things: noticing the expression on a patient's face during a dressing change, understanding the meaning of the expression for the patient in relation to the meaning of the wound (and perhaps the pain), and adjusting action, changing the pressure or the timing of movements. The thoughtful, small practices and adjustments to practices which may seem insignificant or simple often transform the quality of care for the patient and the ward from adequate to excellent. In fact, the little things are not 'little' at all. They may be commonplace and are often taken for granted by the Sisters, but they are fundamentally important to the patient and to the quality of care. It is through noticing, understanding and acting on both the 'little things' and on the big ones that the Sisters' practices are contextual and relational.

Questions persist concerning the accuracy or 'rightness' of the Sisters' understanding and actions. Do the Sisters improve their understanding and skill as they practise, or do their actions merely continue misconceptions or misunderstandings? In this type of interpretative research, issues of judgement cannot be avoided. Connected to them are issues regarding the expertise of the researcher in the clinical area; these are discussed in Appendix 1. Suffice it to say here, that as an informed but non-expert surgical nurse, I was unable to judge whether or not the Sisters practised with the most up-to-date knowledge or intervened in the most effective way possible. However, I did observe, as did they, the effects of their actions in individual situations and was attuned to discrepancies. Evident amongst all of the Sisters was their openness to re-evaluating their own knowledge and practice. They were as open to receiving information from junior nurses as they were from senior consultants and the research literature.

Being attuned to the 'little things', on a moment-by-moment basis, the Sisters seem continually to extend and refine their understanding, and the ways in which they notice and act. They continually keep their practice in question and appear to be in a continual dialogue (not always verbal) with their practice and fellow practitioners.

With the continuing emphasis on the importance of ensuring a systematic approach to decision-making and the planning of nursing care

(McFarlane & Castledine 1982, Brunner & Suddarth 1992), the question is inevitably raised, 'how does the process of noticing, understanding and acting relate to the nursing process?'. Just as the stages of the nursing process might describe any problem-solving process, so noticing, understanding and acting might describe any process of practising. The context, intention and knowing of the nurse are needed in order that the process depicted is that of practising nursing. However, unlike the nursing process, which is usually described as a staged or circular process in which the activities are performed in sequential order, the Sisters notice, understand and act virtually simultaneously. They engage in this process even while they may be systematically planning nursing care in a broader sense. Recent criticisms of the nursing process in that its rational deliberation does not reflect the actual planning and decision-making processes of experienced nurses (cf. Benner & Tanner 1987, Benner et al 1992) are supported in this study. The Sisters' decision-making could be said to be characterized by the intertwined, frequently intuitive process of noticing, understanding and acting.

Thus far I have suggested that everyday experience is more complex, yet more subtle than it is usually given to be. It is not static, but it is linked to ongoing practices and through them with time. Practising and experiencing have the same non-linear temporal character. There is a continual interplay of the past, the present and the future in ongoing practising. It would appear that the Sisters become 'experienced' and develop expertise by being attuned to experience. Being attuned to experience is constituted by an inextricably intertwined process of noticing, understanding and acting which is made possible through a stance of involvement and care. For the Sisters, noticing, understanding and acting is the process of ongoing practising, and as well the process of experiencing. This process cannot be adequately understood unless there is appropriate recognition of the character of knowing which is in practice and is developed through being attuned to experience.

Knowing-in-practice

By focusing attention on taken-for-granted, everyday experience, we have seen its complexity and interconnection with ongoing practising. The Sisters are seen to practise confidently, smoothly, thoughtfully and expertly. Consultants, patients and other nurses have confidence in their practice and knowledge; they continually teach junior staff about patients and how to care for them; they handle a wide range of complex situations, tailoring their practices to the situation. The Sisters' moment-by-moment practice indicates that they are knowledgeable practitioners, continually deepening, refining and extending their knowledge by being attuned to experience. The knowledge they are extending in their everyday practice is, I would suggest, knowing-in-practice.

It may be recalled that in Chapter 2, I made distinctions between theoretical, or formal, knowledge and practical knowledge. I argued there, and in Appendix 1, that conventionally, knowledge and practice are understood to be two separate entities which may be joined together or integrated. I suggested that studying everyday practices from a viewpoint that looks beneath this subject/object, knowing/behaving separation, would enable the relational and contextual nature of experience and practice to be revealed. As we have seen, the process of noticing, understanding and acting was identified, as was the knowing which is already there in the Sisters' taken-for-granted, everyday practices.

In this study, nursing practices have been seen to be ongoing, in the background. They constitute the Sisters' everyday, pragmatic activity and language. These practices make the Sisters' actions count as nursing. Everyday practices cannot be understood as actions consciously performed by intentional actors, nor can they be understood as activities in a behavioural world. Likewise, this multitude of background practices and meanings cannot be isolated or extracted in the form of theoretical formulations or knowledge, even 'background knowledge'. Indeed, this everyday, taken-for-granted level of pragmatic activity 'cannot be understood as *knowledge* at all' (Dreyfus 1983). Practices cannot be considered rote actions, but neither can they be thought of as knowledge per se. That is not to say, however, that knowing is absent from practice. Practices could well be considered to be knowledgeable actions in and of a specific context.

In Chapter 2, the distinction between theoretical knowledge (knowing-that) and practical knowledge (knowing-how) was discussed. Theoretical knowledge is commonly set up as the antithesis of practical knowledge: theoretical, or formal, knowledge is abstract and decontextualized; practical knowledge is always in and of a context. In discussions of knowledge in nursing, practical knowledge is overlooked completely (e.g. Meleis 1991) or accorded less emphasis (e.g. Chinn & Kramer 1995) than theoretical knowledge. It could well be argued that the only recognized form of knowledge within academic nursing circles is theoretical knowledge.

In the conventional view, it has been argued, theoretical knowledge is seen to be separate from practice. Practice, in this view, is usually understood to be something of a behavioural world or an arena of action. Professional practice (cf. Schön 1983) consists of performance in a range of professional situations and the preparation for performance. A central question within this view concerns the process through which theory can be integrated with practice. It is usually proposed in this conventional, albeit ideal view, that nurses should work from a 'scientific' base, using practice theory. Theory, which develops through research, would guide practice by identifying the focus, the means and the goals of practice (Meleis 1991, p 22).

It would follow that, if theoretical knowledge is used in practice, then theory should be discernable in practice. Taking the conception of theory to consist in or be 'represented by the general form of explanation of a number of cognate events or phenomena', Clark (1991) suggests that if theory is to be considered as being used or applied by practitioners, then it must be capable of clear explication and be identified in practice.

... theory in its abstract form must always be discernible to at least one observer if it is ever to be identified as a theory, and the explanations be understood as other than an accidental series of similarities. (p 37)

In this study of the Sisters' everyday experience, it was impossible to discern theoretical knowledge or theory in an abstract form from observations of their practice, or from their accounts. However, that does not mean that the Sisters do not have knowledge of theory or may not have originally learned some of their practice with the help of theoretical knowledge. Essentially, theoretical knowledge which they might once have had in the abstract form is no longer decontextualized and atemporal: it is embedded in the practical context. It has become part of knowing-in-practice. Indeed, theoretical knowledge is only visible in many situations because the Sisters are having to either explain or account for their practices. Even in these circumstances, knowing is seldom, if ever, expressed as acontextual, atemporal theory. The knowing only has its particular meaning because of the context.

Two approaches which run somewhat counter to the prevailing view that theory directs practice are offered by Schön (1983, 1987) and Freidson (1986). They both acknowledge the effect of the context of practice on the practitioner's knowledge. However, the inability to discern theoretical knowledge in the Sisters' practices suggests that Schön's (1987) argument that professionals operate from the basis of an interpersonal theory-in-use is insufficient for explaining the configuration of knowing and practice in particular situations. The Sisters' practices do not appear to emanate from a theory, be it tacit or explicit. To suggest that they do negates the importance of the context in forming (and transforming) knowing.

In his discussion of the reflective practitioner, Schön (1983) proposes the concept of knowing-in-action, which he uses interchangeably with the term, knowing-in-practice. His concept of knowing-in-practice/knowing-in-action differs markedly from the notion of knowing-in-practice in this study. Schön's concept refers to the knowing of the regularities within all of a practitioner's practice, his 'repertoire of expectations, images, and techniques'. He suggests that the practitioner possesses this knowledge and uses it in the action world. This subjectively-held body of knowledge can become increasingly tacit, spontaneous, and automatic; when it does, Schön suggests, the practitioner can 'overlearn', and become selectively inattentive to phenomena that do not fit the categories of his knowing-in-action (Schön 1983 pp 60–61). The categorization of knowing-in-action suggests that it is a form of subjectively-held knowledge which is used as a template in action situations.

Even though Freidson (1986) recognizes the importance of the context, his suggestion that theoretical knowledge is transformed into working knowledge is useful but flawed. Freidson uses Kennedy's (1983) notion of working knowledge, an organized body of knowledge which is subjectively held and used in practice. This approach, like Schön's, however, maintains the separation of the knowing person and the world of practice. This separation was not found in my study. The Sisters' ongoing, taken-for-granted practices were not found to be separate from themselves, nor separate from the specific contexts in which they happened: their practices both formed the situation and were formed by the situation. Much of the time, the Sisters could not be said to 'hold' and 'use' knowledge: their knowing was already in their practices.

The Sisters' knowing-in-practice was found to be similar to practical knowledge, which Dreyfus (1980) suggests can be identified in everyday practical activity. However, it is proposed that there is a subtle but important difference between knowing-in-practice and practical knowledge. For the purposes of clarity and illustration, practical knowledge is usually set in stark opposition to theoretical knowledge. This is understandable, given the elusiveness of practical knowledge and the concomitant difficulty in creating an adequate depiction of it. Practical knowledge, it was suggested in Chapter 2, has been variously described as intuition, embodied intelligence or practices (Dreyfus & Dreyfus 1986). The conceptual inconsistency of Benner's (1984) six areas of practical knowledge further illustrates the difficulty of describing practical knowledge. I would like to suggest, however, that while the delineation between practical knowledge and theoretical knowledge may be a useful and necessary one, treating them in a dichotomous

manner does not adequately deal with their interconnection in the midst of ongoing practising. This interconnection in practice is best characterized as knowing-in-practice.

In their everyday practices, the Sisters did not seem to be using theory as Benner suggests, to tell them 'where to look for legitimate concerns and what constitutes legitimacy' (Benner & Wrubel 1989 p 20) but theory was not absent from their practices. As the Sisters took on board formal, theoretical knowledge, the contextualization of that knowledge by means of their practical knowing created new knowing-in-practice.

In most of their everyday practices, the Sisters' formal knowledge was hidden, like the brandy in a brandy fruitcake which can be tasted but cannot be extracted in its pure form, the form in which it went into the mixture. Like the brandy in the fruitcake, formal knowledge is only a small part of the whole of everyday practice. Also like the brandy, it is transformed in practice from something separate and discrete to something which is united with its context. Formal knowledge is not transformed, however, into a kind of static knowledge. The Sisters' knowing is specific to a situation and is revealed through the situation. As the situation changes, on a minute-by-minute basis, so does the configuration of knowledge, and indeed the character of knowing. In responding to the needs of patients and the demands of the situation, the Sister may extend and create new ways of knowing in noticing, understanding and acting.

The evidence in this study suggests that in day-by-day, moment-by-moment practice, the knowing with which the Sisters practise expertly, the knowing which characterizes the quality of their noticing, understanding and acting and which develops by being attuned to experience can be called *knowing-in-practice*. The Sisters' knowing-in-practice is imbued with theory and practical knowing, but it is knowing in a context: theory cannot readily be discerned. Already a part of everyday, ongoing pragmatic activity and informed by theoretical knowing, knowing-in-practice is, at the same time, more subtle and encompassing than the separate notions of theory and practice. Theoretical knowledge and practical knowing are already integrated in practice.

Developing knowing-in-practice

In the same way that the Sisters' knowing-in-practice develops, so does their capacity to notice, understand and act in ways tailored to the individual patient and the ward. I have suggested that knowing-in-practice develops by being attuned to experience. Being attuned to experience is an ongoing thoughtful, complex, multifaceted, reflexive and reflective process through which the Sister herself grows and changes as her practice develops: she becomes 'experienced'. This happens, as it has already been said, during moment-by-moment, day-by-day practising with patients and others on the ward (and outwith the ward). Before moving onto a more abstract level, it may be useful to look at some features of the Sisters' experience through which their knowing-in-practice was encouraged and enhanced.

As might be expected, for all of the Sisters, the patients emerge as the primary source of learning about clinical care. From the patients they learn about illness, the process of recovery, the meaning of being ill and the effects of their own practices. Patients are the most meaningful constituent of the Sisters' milieu[1].

Common to all of the Sisters is a confidence about their abilities to notice, and a sureness of action. Confidence does not just arise from developing knowing-in-practice, it also enables its development. Because of their confidence, the Sisters are able to act in situations, which in turn present opportunities for developing new ways of noticing, understanding and acting. Their confidence also inspires others and sets up opportunities for new experience. Although they are confident in their understanding of a wide range of situations, the Sisters are not complacent and they consistently keep their practice and their understandings open to question. They confirm and extend their understanding, their actions and how they notice through a process which is much like a dialogue with their own practice. This dialogue is part of being attuned to their own and to others' experience.

Important to all of the Sisters are times in their experience when they were given responsibility with concomitant support from doctors, ward sisters or staff nurses. Having responsibility with support seems to be a key to developing confidence. It engages the nurse in the situation and engenders the commitment and involvement required to take action which, in turn, opens new ways of noticing and understanding. A particularly important time for most of the Sisters to have responsibility with support was as senior students or in their first staff nurse position. The role of responsibility in spurring-on learning is also a recurrent theme in research on learning in everyday experience in other fields (Burgoyne & Hodgson 1983, McCall et al 1988, Van Velsor & Hughes 1990, Rossing 1991). Exploring the meaning of having responsibility with support at different times in nurses' careers would seem fruitful, particularly with the introduction of new educational programmes such as the 1992 Programmes in the United Kingdom[2].

These features of the Sisters' experience point towards the relational and contextual nature of being attuned to experience. Learning occurs in the midst of practising, in the midst of experiencing.

It was suggested that in the conventional view, theory is derived from systematic observations of practice, or developed outwith the practice milieu and then matched to, or applied in, practice situations by nurses. The corollary of this view is that, in order to improve practice, the nurses should reflect on their experiences, bringing theory into this re-examination. In reflection, the nurses would not only gain a new perspective but would also acquire new theoretical knowledge which could be applied in practice.

Conventional discussions of learning from experience mirror those on integrating theory and practice. Experience and learning are held to be separate entities, awaiting connection through a process in which action and reflection are in some sort of a dialectical, staged or circular relationship. In the reflection phase of experiential learning models, individuals reflect on entities which somehow have been abstracted from periods of experience or action. Through these processes, new theoretical formulations are created, and then tested out in new experiences. This feature, common to all of these models, overlooks three things which have been found in this study:

1. Ongoing practice is imbued with the thinking characterized by Clark (1991) as 'the fluid, unlogical, intuitive, expressive and erratic character of ordinary thinking and problem-solving'.
2. People are experiencing all the time, including during times of reflection.
3. Knowing-in-practice can be extended and developed without even reaching conscious awareness.

This last point, the extension and development of knowing-in-practice in the midst of everyday taken-for-granted experiencing is perhaps where this study differs most from other studies which address the extension and development of practice knowledge. This takes us back to Heidegger's doorknob. Unlike other studies (e.g. Benner 1984), which suggest that experience happens when the doorknob sticks and there is an active refinement of preconceived notions and expectations about the nature of doorknobs, this study has found that the Sisters are experiencing all the time. Even when the doorknob does not stick, every time they open a door their hands feel the doorknob and gradually, over time, they come to feel what normal doorknobs feel like and how easily or stiffly doorknobs turn. Thus, when the doorknob sticks, experience has already given them scales upon which to weigh 'stuck-ness'. While the doorknob provides a simple example, the Sisters, I would suggest, become attuned to such things as the sounds of a ward, the look of pain and the smell of wounds through a similar process.

The suggestion that some knowing-in-practice develops imperceptibly raises questions about how practitioners' ways of working are depicted. For instance, Clark (1991) proposes the following in respect of practitioners in community and social work:

I have described the practitioners' way of working as practical theorising. While being obviously practical in character, this process does also merit the appellation 'theorising' because it entails classification, the search for patterns and regularities, and above all the business of practically adequate explanation and prediction. It partakes therefore of the essential characteristics of theoretical knowledge. It is emphatically not the mechanical application of inert facts, but represents the intelligent use of complex and disparate knowledge at all levels. (Clark 1991 p 156)

This idea of searching, connecting and making sense of regularities (and appreciating differences) in everyday practising, which Clark names practical theorizing, is similar to what Benner calls extending knowledge through interpretative theory. It is explaining in a way which attends to the local, particular, and specific whilst maintaining the meanings in context (Benner & Wrubel 1989). She suggests that expert nursing practitioners work in this way. I would agree that the Sisters do work in this way a great deal of the time, but not all of the time. That is not to say that they do not practise expertly; rather, it is to say that practical theorizing does not completely describe how the Sisters work.

Benner & Wrubel go on to suggest that practice and theory can exist in a dialogical relationship. In this relationship, theory frames the questions and guides the practitioner where to look and what to ask, whilst clinical practice, because of its complexity and variety, is itself an arena of knowledge development. Both Clark and Benner & Wrubel rightly propose a different relationship between theory and practice, one in which practice is primary. However, to use the word 'theorizing' to describe what practitioners do, is not without its problems. The word theory is usually associated with academic and formal knowledge. While there may be benefits to using it to describe practitioner action, there is a risk that the word may inadvertently bring with it the conventional associations and expectations of theoretical knowledge. This is of particular concern if it perpetuates the understanding that the scales with which knowledge is to be weighed must be those of formal or theoretical knowledge. What is unique about knowing-in-practice may be obscured.

Surgical nursing, because of its inherently practical and kinesic nature (the 'disparate knowledge at all levels'), includes a good proportion of knowing 'in the fingertips' and understanding the meanings of fine gradations in smells and sounds. Neither term, practical theorizing nor interpretative theory, normally brings such knowing to mind. So much taken for granted, this knowing does not often come into descriptions of 'experiences' or 'paradigm cases'. It begins and remains tacit, ineffable and intuitive. It is 'absorbed' or 'picked up' in ongoing experiencing. By being attuned, the Sisters develop knowing that can be articulated and described; by being attuned, they develop bodily knowing that is tacit and intuitive.

Being attuned to experience encompasses both reflection and action. It is not atheoretical, but the complexity of experience suggests that knowing-in-practice is developed in a number of ways. By separating experience and learning, such as happens in experiential learning models and models of reflection, the ongoing 'picking up', continual comparison and dialogue with practice which can occur in the midst of ongoing experience in practice is omitted from the under-standing of learning. Being attuned to experience points towards this ongoing reflexiveness in everyday experiencing.

THE PRIMACY OF EVERYDAY EXPERIENCE IN PRACTICE

This study began from a concern that there was something happening in nurses' everyday experience which not only enabled them to care for patients, but also contributed to the devel-opment of expertise. Upon examination, the taken-for-granted practice and experiences of 'excellent, experienced' Ward Sisters, were found to be rich, complex and imbued with theoretical and practical knowledge. Through the process of practising — noticing, understanding and acting — which stems from a stance of involvement and care, the Sisters are attuned to experience and continually develop their knowing-in-practice. They are learning all the time. This study shows the wealth of knowledge with which the Sisters practise and how important being attuned to everyday experience is to its ongoing development.

Thinking of everyday practising as a process in which nurses can continually broaden and deepen knowing-in-practice, opens the way to thinking of the nurse as a 'knowledge worker'. Until recently, nursing has not been thought of as a cognate discipline. Witness the difficulty nursing has experienced in gaining a secure place in higher education in the United Kingdom and other countries, and the length of time it has taken the profession to formally recognize the role of knowledge in practice. For example, the United Kingdom has only recently identified that the new practitioner would be 'a knowledgeable doer' (UKCC 1986). If we are to understand the nurse to be a 'knowledge worker' then a much broader sense of knowledge must be contemplated.

At present, the legitimate knowledge in nursing curricula is formal knowledge, with knowing-in-practice relegated to informal discussions on the ward or as a subordinate part of theory courses. This is no less the case in North America (Diekelmann et al 1989) than it is in Scotland (P Darbyshire, personal communication, 1990). Hiding real-life nursing knowledge behind the accounts of formal knowledge has served to 'eclipse' many aspects of nursing practice (Campbell & Jackson 1992). This state of affairs is due, in part, to the fact that nursing has not systematically engaged in the development of clinical knowledge through 'documenting, con-serving, and enhancing the unique knowledge of the experienced clinician . . .' (Benner & Wrubel 1982). To realize the primacy of practice, clinical knowledge has to be systematically developed.

If knowing-in-practice is to be captured, everyday situations in nursing need to be written down. Writing puts practice in an enduring public space. Descriptions of everyday nursing practices would include their temporal nature, the particulars and the mixture of thinking and doing. Even though only a fraction of the richness and nuances of practice can ever be communicated, writing about practice in narrative form reveals far more than the skeletal form of theoretical knowledge.

In an oral culture such as nursing, clinicians are frequently not used to writing about their practice. If the Sisters in this study are any indication, nurses are not even used to talking about their taken-for-granted practice in detail. And, as this research shows, much of nursing practice will not be communicated in writing, or told about as memorable experiences in interviews. It is passed on in gesture, precept or by incidental conversation to junior nurses. If this knowing is to be captured, innovative approaches may need to be devised. However, the fact that knowing-in-practice is often ephemeral does not diminish its importance.

A powerful rationale for encouraging experienced nurses to name and describe their taken-for-granted practices is that the process brings hidden practices and knowledge to light. Although knowing about them may not prompt nurses to change their practices, they sometimes gain a new appreciation of how they work. They can then point out these invisible practices and knowing to junior nurses. In this way, experienced nurses are better able to help junior nurses notice salient aspects of a situation, make comparisons and links and explore new ways of acting.

The language about everyday experience in nursing practice, as well as opportunities for talking about it, need to be enhanced. Until nurses can accurately and readily depict their practice, there is a danger that nursing practice will continue to be overlooked and undervalued. As Attridge & Callahan (1989) point out, nurses themselves must develop pride in their work. In order to be proud of their work, 'nurses must understand, describe, and come to value what they believe and do' (p 62). If nurses do not fully recognize the value of their own work, others most certainly will not accord it sufficient worth.

The contribution of nursing care to patient outcomes is increasingly acknowledged even though the complexity of nursing care and the difficulty in assessing patient outcomes make it hard to make direct links between the two. Nevertheless, as hospital environments grow more dependent upon documentary evidence, the ability to articulate nursing practice is critical. If nursing practices remain invisible, clinical nurses and nursing managers cannot bring them into discussions at decision-making tables, nor can they be brought into the formation of measurements and descriptors of nursing work.

There is a well-founded concern that much of the substance of nursing practice is being overlooked and undervalued in current organizational change strategies. An increasing number of hospitals are undergoing workplace re-engineering

or restructuring, a process that is largely data driven (Hammer & Champy 1993). Within restructuring, practices that cannot be reduced to discrete data bits are frequently accorded less value, because the focus of attention remains on tasks and processes that can be articulated and measured. As a result of the need for measurement, practices change to fit in with organization and documentation requirements and important aspects of nurses' work can become obscured (Campbell 1984, Campbell & Jackson 1992).

Practices and processes that cannot be well articulated or do not fit into measurement or documentation requirements are not always accorded their true value, despite their important link to patient outcome. As McWilliam & Wong (1994) aptly show, a great deal of nursing's indirect contribution to patient care remains overlooked and unrecognized. The qualitative, intangible elements of nursing practice do impact care outcomes. There is a danger that if much of nursing work continues to be hidden, hospital and health care restructuring and reorganization may result in an erosion of nursing practice with a concomitant change in patient outcome. In order to bring the value of nursing practice to the wider public, it is imperative that nurses learn to communicate the complexity and character of the crucial, yet often taken-for-granted, 'little things' of everyday nursing work.

RETHINKING OUR UNDERSTANDING OF EXPERIENCE AND LEARNING

This research has shown that nurses learn and deepen their knowing and expertise in the midst of everyday practice through being attuned to experience. If nurses are to be understood as 'knowledge workers', then the range of approaches which can be taken to develop ways of knowing must be acknowledged: from formal inquiry, to practical theorizing, to picking-up and absorbing. If the complexity and range of nurses' knowledge and everyday experience are recognized and valued, then the different ways of being attuned to experience have a better chance of being acknowledged.

The development of knowledge has conventionally been thought to be the province of researchers and higher education. Usually in nursing programmes, theory is taught in the college or school and the student, the integrator of theory and practice, is expected to apply it in the practice situation (Alexander 1980, Melia 1987). Alternative approaches are being developed in some problem-based learning curricula, in practice-driven approaches to curricula (MacLeod 1995) and in some nursing staff development programmes (Dick 1983). Such alternative approaches systematically provide relevant theory to students and practising nurses in the clinical area to augment their knowing-in-practice. Instead of theory being provided in a form most suitable for teaching, it is provided where and when it is needed for learning. The Sisters are, in fact, doing this informally as they help students learn to care for patients. If practice and knowing-in-practice are indeed at the centre of nursing, then educational programmes need to reconsider where and when theory would most fruitfully be available to enhance the development of knowing-in-practice.

This study suggests that experience spans all situations. Being attuned to experience, the Sisters act, understand and notice, comparing similarities and differences in their own understanding and experiences, no matter where they occur. The notion of 'transfer of learning' (cf. Alexander 1980, Bigge 1982), which has arisen as a way of making a theoretical bridge between theory and practice situations for learners, is cast in a new light. Rather than being an issue of generalizability, knowing across situations may hinge instead on the ability of nurses to recognize similar aspects among different contexts, understand their meaning, make comparisons and connections, and have the confidence to act.

The importance of recognizing experience in everyday practice has special relevance for the ongoing development of clinical nurses. Although current plans for continuing education (e.g. UKCC 1990) acknowledge the need to legitimate experienced nurses' already-held knowledge, there are still few higher education courses for experienced nurses that are designed to strengthen clinical know-how. Most courses presuppose clinical knowledge and focus on the addition of theoretical knowledge. I suggest that another approach is required, one in which the clinical knowing-in-practice of experienced nurses is acknowledged and enhanced. In such a programme, experienced nurses would have the opportunity to engage in a dialogue about their own practice, bringing theoretical knowledge into the conversation of practice[3], rather than the other way around.

Some of the approaches in this study could be used in such a programme. The study has provided the Sisters with several important opportunities to engage in conversations about their practice. In the course of the study the Sisters have had the opportunity to: describe their everyday experiences; be listened and attended to; have their practices witnessed; see and comment on interpretations of their own and others' practice; meet with others to share experiences in practice; most particularly, to converse with others of the same level of experience and skill. They have been able to gain new perspectives on their practice: new links have been made and new dialogues opened with others and with their own practices. The conversation is about practising nursing and being attuned to experience. Through the conversation, naming one's own practices and seeing them legitimated can be a confidence-boosting and empowering experience[4].

It has been well argued by Campbell (1984) and Street (1992) that in the face of organizational practices, including documentary practices, that serve to structure nursing work, it is not enough simply to begin the conversation. Nurses need to undertake more systematic processes of reflection and collaborative critique of taken-for-granted practices and the context within which they practice. I would suggest that such reflection and critique can happen only when nurses begin to name, explore and celebrate the knowing in their everyday practices and experience. Naming nursing practices is not just a matter of identifying and communicating the practices. In developing a language that clearly speaks of the situated nature of nursing practice, the practices themselves are re-created. As Usher (1992) says, 'Language regulates and forms experience rather than simply being a device for naming it' (p 208). From a base of re-creating practices in the discourse of nursing, nurses will be better placed to act as collaborators with managers, patients and other health care providers in changing structures and practices for improved care. Explorations of nursing experience can serve as the basis for interpretative action projects in which nurses examine and change their caring practices and work structures.

My suggestions for exploring nursing experience shed new light on the current enthusiasm for reflective practice in nursing. In this and earlier chapters, I have pointed out the limitations of current understandings of reflection and have shown that being attuned to experience encompasses both reflection and action. James & Clarke (1994) among others, identify the considerable problems inherent in the notion of reflective practice. Perhaps the most problematic use of reflective practice in nursing is where nursing practices are understood not as background, taken-for-granted practices that both form and are formed by the situation, but as something held individually by nurses that are amenable to reconfiguration by cognitive, reflective activity. In this view the conversation of nursing practice moves from one of collective experience and understanding to a more limited one of subjectively-held experience in an objective world. A more productive conversation would include approaching reflection in nursing practice and education in a way that fully acknowledges the situated nature of nursing practice, experience, knowing and learning.

The approaches suggested here have a different focus and goal than do the management-directed approaches of the learning organization (Senge 1990, Watkins & Marsick 1993). Unlike the learning organization, the goal is not productivity and the focus is not the engineering of systematic organizational change. My research suggests that when nurses engage in a process of interpreting their everyday experience and practice, empower-

ment can follow. The structuring or direct facilitation of learning takes the agenda for learning and practice out of the nurses' own hands. When nurses are given opportunities to name their practices and uncover and extend their knowing-in-practice they will take the agenda in ways that improve the care of their patients and their own working lives. As Attridge & Callahan (1989) have found, it is control over their work situations that lends satisfaction to nurses' working lives. Nurses rarely seek power for themselves, but 'almost always for patient or group advancement' (p 55). When organizations seek to harness and facilitate incidental learning in the name of developing a learning organization, questions about interests, goals and power are unavoidable.

Rather than suggesting specific ways in which the knowing-in-practice of experienced nurses can be valued and enhanced, it may be more productive to suggest where the discussion on nursing practice and experience might go next. At the risk of oversimplification, it is my observation that when clinical nursing practice development is discussed in America, discussion often centres at the level of the specific nurse and her skills: responses to problems are individualized. In the United Kingdom, discussion often centres at the organizational level: what structures might be most useful to ensure standards, educational programmes or clinical advancement. This research demonstrates that to recognize and value knowing-in-practice while enhancing the process of being attuned to experience, a middle approach is needed: an approach that acknowledges the practising of individuals in an organization. Fruitful discussions would centre on ways of re-shaping the professional and organizational structures, including ongoing managerial and educational strategies, to enable nurses, individually and collectively, to develop excellence in everyday clinical practice. In order for these discussions to be successful, there must be adequate recognition of nurses' everyday experience in practice and its contribution to the development of nursing and health care.

Notes

[1] There is a growing body of literature about the important role of knowing the patient in providing quality nursing care (Jenny & Logan 1992, MacLeod 1993, Tanner et al 1993). It is perhaps not surprising that at the same time as knowing the patient is a key to good nursing care, so patients are the main source of learning for the nurse.

[2] Formerly known as Project 2000.

[3] I am indebted to Nancy Diekelmann and Steve Tilley who, from different beginnings, are also exploring this notion of the conversation of nursing practice. See in particular, Tilley (1995).

[4] The approaches suggested here were incorporated into a practice-driven, phenomenological approach to an Introduction to Nursing course in a 4-year undergraduate nursing curriculum in which practising nurses helped first-year students explore what it means to be a nurse, what it means to care and what it meant to be a person or family receiving care. See MacLeod & Farrell (1994), MacLeod (1995) and Wilkinson et al (1995).
See also Benner (1991) for her discussion of narratives of learning.

Appendix 1

Research approach and methods

INTRODUCTION

The approach taken in this study lies within the interpretative tradition, a tradition which seeks to understand meaning in human experience. The particular form of an interpretative study is determined by a number of factors. Among them are: the particular strand of the interpretative tradition which informs the study; the nature of the substantive concern; the contingencies of the research situation; the capacities and inclinations of the researcher. More specifically, this study has been informed by hermeneutic phenomenology, a strand of the interpretative tradition which follows Heidegger's (1962) ontological turn. The everyday experience of surgical ward sisters, as expressed in their accounts and observed in their ongoing practice, provided the material for interpretation.

In this qualitative form of research, the researcher is far from invisible. More than just a 'research instrument' (Sanday 1979, Guba & Lincoln 1981), the researcher is influential in all stages of the study. Inevitably then, my own experiences and skills have been drawn upon, tested and extended through this study. Their influence on the course of the research will be discussed throughout this account. Before moving to the specifics of the research method, however, it may be useful to give a brief overview of the central themes in the interpretative tradition as well as the particular perspective afforded by hermeneutic phenomenology.

THE INTERPRETATIVE APPROACH

The interpretative tradition can be traced to Dilthey, who first attempted to create a distinctive method for the human sciences by proposing that understanding has its roots in the process of human life itself. According to Dilthey, in the course of everyday life we humans have to make sense of the situations we are in, so we can act accordingly. These acts of understanding *(Verstehen)*, which are lived by us, constitute our 'lived experience' *(Erlebnis)*. In turn, the manifestations of human life (words, gestures or actions), what Dilthey called the various forms of 'life expression' *(Lebensäusserung)*, point back towards lived experience as their source. Hence, for Dilthey, and then Weber, the understanding sought by social scientists referred to a deep level of comprehension, involving capturing the expressions of 'inner realities' (Giddens 1982). It can be seen then, that central to this notion of *Verstehen*, is grasping the subjective meaning of a person's action from the actor's point of view.

Husserl's foundational work provided Dilthey with a phenomenological viewpoint from which to develop his hermeneutics for the social sciences (Mueller-Vollmer 1985). Within Husserl's philosophy, phenomenology was a means for seeking a solid foundation for knowledge by analysing consciousness and its objects in direct experience. He proposed that all forms of knowledge have their roots in consciousness: consciousness is intentional, that is, it is consciousness of something. Husserl argued that, in our direct experience of the world, we suspend our presupposition of an object's reality; we constitute matter/objects in our consciousness of them. This process, of stepping into a philosophical attitude, of distancing oneself from commonly-held understanding about the phenomenon in question, Husserl called 'bracketing'. Bracketing our presuppositions about objects of consciousness allows us to come at phenomena freshly — to examine them as they are constituted in our mental content. This concentration on subjective experience is at the heart of Husserl's work. Both Dilthey and Husserl, continuing the philosophical tradition of Descartes, understood humans to be subjects in an object world: '... spectators, observers, separated by an invisible plate-glass window from the world of objects in which we find ourselves' (Magee 1987 p 258).

This distinction between subjective experience and the object world has been maintained in various strands of the, by no means coherent, interpretative tradition which has been highly influenced by the work of Dilthey and Husserl. Among the most influential approaches in nursing and education have been social phenomenology (Berger & Luckmann 1967, Schutz & Luckmann 1974), ethnomethodology (Garfinkel 1967), and the symbolic interactionist approaches of Mead (1934) and Blumer (1969). These divergent approaches, while having considerably different views of experience, meaning, and the nature of the person and his or her context, nevertheless consider the person and the world to be separate though closely interrelated entities. The phenomenological tradition, largely shaped by Husserl's work, and sometimes described as a descriptive approach (Spiegelberg 1982, Omery 1983, Munhall & Oiler Boyd 1993), is represented for the most part in studies in nursing and education by the approach taken by Giorgi (1975, 1985) and van Kaam (1959), among others. This approach has concentrated on providing rich descriptions of people's subjective experiences.

As we have seen in Chapters 2 and 3, the studies in nursing and education which have been based on these approaches have provided a wealth of information about the experiences of learners, the world of learning, and specific aspects of nurses' experience in practice. However, it could be fairly said that some of the studies' shortcomings could be traced to the studies' philosophical underpinnings. These shortcomings include the inability to adequately capture the complexity of nursing practice, the inability to grasp ongoing experiencing as well as past experience, and the oversight of the inseparability of the person and his or her context. As noted in Chapters 2 and 3, these shortcomings are not as pronounced in the interpretative studies which followed the turn in phenomenology taken by Heidegger (Gray-Snelgrove 1982, Diekelmann 1992, 1993, Benner 1984, 1994, Darbyshire 1994).

The phenomenological turn taken by Heidegger and augmented by Gadamer and Ricoeur points the researcher not only towards a different approach to analysing the research material, but also towards a different focus of concern in field-work. The central, relevant themes in Heidegger's major work, *Being and Time* (Heidegger 1962) are explored next.

Hermeneutic phenomenology

Heidegger, himself drawing on Dilthey and Husserl, proposed that the questions they were pursuing about how people *know*, were only secondary to a consideration of how people *are* in their everyday endeavours. If one looks beneath to the human situation, it does not appear to be a situation in which a conscious, autonomous subject is directing one's mind to mental representations of the world. While we may consciously direct our minds towards objects, it is only possible because we are already beings who are coping in the world. This irreducible connection between being and the world is reflected in Heidegger's starting point, which is not the separate person or subject, but is rather *Dasein* which, roughly translated, means existence or 'being-there'.

Dasein is not seen as a conscious subject, a self-contained source of meaning-giving consciousness, but as an individual dependent upon shared, taken-for-granted, background practices for the content of life and for all meaning and intelligibility. That is because '*Dasein* always understands itself in terms of its existence' (Heidegger 1962, p 33). In *Being and Time*, Heidegger explores these ways of Being. What is notable about the ways of Being of *Dasein* is that they are all ways of comporting, of being-in-the-world.

The 'world' for Heidegger is not an impersonal, objective world, but rather is closer to a personal world which cannot be conceived as separate from the self. Heidegger shows in his phenomenological analysis of *Dasein* that there is no subject-object delineation prior to knowledge of the self in the world. Neither can there be knowledge of the world as being present without the self. Our world, Heidegger proposes, is made up of background practices, social practices and historical contexts. It is unobtrusive, presupposed and is usually transparent to us. Heidegger says that we dwell in the world — we inhabit it. When we inhabit something, it becomes part of us and pervades our relation to other objects in the world (Dreyfus 1991). In this way, for instance, we inhabit our language. We are at home in it and relate to other people and objects through it.

In the same way that the world is unobtrusive, so are our tools and the practices that we under-take without thought. Heidegger proposes that people have three distinct yet interrelated modes of engagement, or involvement, with objects in their world: ready-to-hand, unready-to-hand and present-at-hand. In the ready-to-hand mode, people are actively engaged in practical projects — objects are taken for granted. There is no conscious awareness of the activities as separate events or parts. There is unthinking, holistic awareness, a concernful absorption. Common, everyday practices are taken for granted — they are so familiar. Only when there is an inter-ruption or problem in the smooth flow of activity, does the person disengage from this mode.

Meeting a problem or experiencing an inter-ruption in the smooth flow of practical activity, and moving to an awareness of the problem is the mode of unready-to-hand. The breakdown of action is noticed, it becomes salient, but our noticing of it remains within the context of the background of activity in which we are engaged.

We enter the present-at-hand mode when we step back from involved activity to reflect upon it. The ready-at-hand phenomena in the world which previously we did not see, are brought into view through the mode of presence-at-hand (Heidegger 1962).

Although the social world is not specifically addressed as such in *Being and Time*, *Dasein* is already socialized into background skills and cultural knowledge. From birth, we live and learn within practices that contain an interpretation of what it is to be human in our culture. Thus, we learn what it is to be a person within our historical, cultural and social context. As well as learning what it is to be, we learn what an object is, how objects are to be used and how we are to relate to them. Our understandings of what it is to be human fit together with what it is to be an object. Both are aspects of a more general understanding of Being within a particular culture (Dreyfus 1991). Rather than being a separate mind, needing connection with other minds, *Dasein* is already being-with others, sharing the background understandings and culture. The shared taken-for-granted background makes understanding possible, but as all of us have differing experiences and differing histories, all is not shared and times of misunderstanding are inevitable.

Before moving on to a discussion of how this approach of hermeneutic phenomenology affected the evolution of the study, specific reference must be made to the notions of understanding and interpretation which inform this study. They are of particular importance because of the concern in this study to uncover what is usually hidden from us, the nature of everyday experience in nursing practice.

Understanding and interpretation

Both 'understanding' and 'interpretation' are words that have specific meanings within Heideggerian phenomenology. For Heidegger, understanding is the power to grasp one's own possibilities for being, within the context of one's world. To use an often quoted example of Heidegger's, the practice of hammering only makes sense in terms of nails, wood, and wooden structures, equipment which Heidegger calls the totality of significance. This relational structure of the world, in turn, is only possible because of the skills, such as holding objects, wearing clothes, walking and moving, which have enabled one to get to the position of hammering. This context of assignments or references — the taken-for-granted background of the world and our capacities for being in the world — is what is disclosed in understanding.

Understanding, for Heidegger, is an ontological

process, a disclosure of what is real for people. It is not merely a conscious or unconscious process.

It is not a special capacity or gift for feeling into the situation of another person, nor is it the power to grasp the meaning of some 'expression of life' on a deeper level. Understanding is conceived not as something to be possessed but rather as a mode or constituent element of being-in-the-world. (Palmer 1969 p 131)

As a central constituent of being-in-the-world, understanding has a temporal sense. According to Heidegger, we are temporal beings. Our temporality shows itself in our ongoing activity and practices. Time could be said to be *in* the activity. Being in a situation, we act from the past, in the ongoing present, but always projected towards the possibilities of the future. Our horizon of understanding, which embodies this temporality, is one of projection. It is explicated through interpretation. Interpretation, in turn, always presupposes meaning and understanding. There is no hope of presuppositionless interpretation. 'In every case this interpretation is grounded in *something we have in advance — in a fore-having*' (Heidegger 1962 p 191). This fore-having is the background of meaning and experience embedded in our practices, language and history. It forms our 'horizon' for interpretation.

Heidegger suggests that interpretation is central to our constitution in the world: *Dasein* is self-interpreting. We understand ourselves in some specific way. 'Dasein is interpretation all the way down' (Dreyfus 1991 p 25). Heidegger contends that this understanding of self is not totally available to us. Our background meanings and pre-understandings, our interpretations of being-in-the-world, are inaccessible to us, concealed through our everyday existence.

Heidegger's example of a hammer illustrates how we only become aware of our practices and the meaning of them when some breakdown occurs. A hammer that is merely present, can be weighed, catalogued and its properties assessed. However, the meaning of the hammer is not disclosed through mere contemplation. A hammer needs to be used to display its aspects in a functional context. When breakdown occurs, when the object moves from being ready-to-hand to unready-to-hand, the meaning of the object or practices are highlighted; they emerge from their everyday background of unobtrusiveness. When the nail does not go in smoothly, the hammer ceases to be a taken-for-granted tool and it may be interpreted as being too heavy for the job at hand.

This example suggests a hermeneutic principle, that through interpretation, the being of something is disclosed when it emerges from the background to the full functional context of the world (Palmer 1969 p 133). Thus, the act of interpretation reveals the relational and contextual nature of being-in-the-world. It is this focus of hermeneutic phenomenology, on disclosing the relational and contextual nature of being-in-the-world through interpretation, which makes it useful for revealing the nature of everyday experience in nursing practice.

Such ostensibly abstract theoretical considerations may seem far removed from the world of nursing practice. Nonetheless, as it will become apparent, they have critical implications for how the study was pursued. They will be seen to lead to an approach which focuses on how the nurses practise in their everyday world of work, and which interprets their practices and experiences in such a way that they are not separated from either the nurses or their ongoing practice situation.

THE STUDY

The goal of the study was to examine the nature of everyday experience in nursing practice and its contribution to the development of clinical expertise. The intention was to come to an understanding of everyday experience among nurses who were considered to be excellent practitioners. To this end, I observed 10 experienced surgical nurses in practice and interviewed them about their experiences. The field notes and interview transcripts provided the 'material', the text for interpretation.

The process and spirit of this research has much in common with the hermeneutic circle, in which we understand something only in relation to its parts, and as we gain knowledge of a part, our understanding of the whole changes (Heidegger 1962). This understanding of research presumes an openness: it is an approach which could be described as a dialogue, hearing what the nurses are saying and doing and, in turn, responding to the questions that are posed by their practice and experience (Gadamer 1979). Thus, the plan of the study was not pre-set, but rather it evolved as a new sense of the parts and the whole emerged.

The study was not formless, however. As I mentioned in Chapter 1, I kept two principles at the forefront throughout. First, my attention was focused on the nurse-in-practice, not on the nurse removed from a context, nor on the context without the nurse. Second, I endeavoured to 'keep close' to experience, to continually ask while in the field and during interpretation, 'What does this mean about experience?'. These two principles were touchstones throughout the study. I considered them to be much like the central agenda when planning an educational conference or programme. I have found that when the central agenda is clear, then there is room to be spontaneous and 'go with the flow'. If the agenda is not focused, if the 'ends-in-view' (Dewey 1925) are unclear, or if the important issues have not been thoroughly thought through then one is too preoccupied with them to be able to appreciate the possibilities for spontaneous action. One is also too preoccupied to know when to deviate from the plan, or when to abandon it altogether.

The focus of my attention throughout this study was the nurse in the context of her experience, specifically her nursing practices. The goal of the research was not to get at the essences of lived experience from the perspective of the nurses, as in other phenomenological research (cf. Oiler

1982, Forrest 1989), nor was it to determine the operative social processes as in other interpretative research (cf. Chenitz & Swanson 1984, 1986, Melia 1987). Rather, in this research I sought to illuminate themes in nursing experience, to discover the relational issues between the nurse and her context and to achieve understanding.

As mentioned earlier, the skills and inclinations of the researcher, though important in all types of research (Polanyi [1958]1962) are of particular importance in interpretative research. Clark (1990) provides a useful discussion of the expertise needed by the interpretative researcher who is attempting to understand the nature of knowing in practice. He rightly suggests that in addition to knowledge of the theoretical area and the tools and techniques of research in the particular discipline, the researcher needs to be accomplished in skills which enable her to comprehend and make sense of taken-for-granted practices and commonsense knowledge. As Giddens (1976 p 155) puts it, 'The social scientist of necessity draws upon the same sorts of skills as those whose conduct he seeks to analyse in order to describe it'.

First amongst these skills is language. It is not enough to understand the words, it is necessary to grasp such things as jokes, allusions and the different meanings of words in different contexts when used by different speakers. The second area is skill in comprehending the meaning of non-verbal behaviour. Although Clark puts this second to language in importance, I would suggest that skills in understanding everyday language and non-verbal behaviour are equally important and inseparable. The third area is knowledge of the disciplines, conventions, ideologies and practices of the particular field, in this case, nursing. The fourth area concerns the relevant contextual knowledge, the knowledge of nursing practice in the wards under study. The fifth concerns skills of the research method: in this study, observation and reflexive interviewing techniques, and hermeneutic interpretation skills. Sixth and last, are the attributes of age, gender and ethnicity. Each of these six areas will be addressed in the subsequent discussion about

how the study was carried out. I hope that by describing my reasons and actions, my mistakes, as well as my successes, will be open to view.

One of the perennial concerns of researchers in the qualitative mode is the issue of rigour. According to Robinson & Thorne (1988 p 74), 'careful reflection, meticulous reporting and vigorous debate must be hallmarks of the process [qualitative researchers] use ...' Guba & Lincoln (1981) suggest that researchers spell out their 'decision trail' so that others may audit the process. At the risk of being overly detailed, I will attempt in this discussion to explain the decisions which I took and indicate how they influenced the course of the study. I hope that this detail may be helpful to other researchers who may be planning a similar study. The first of these decisions concerns the specific research questions.

Guiding questions

At the outset of the study, several specific questions were created to serve as guides for the field work. I began to negotiate access to nurses in the clinical area with the question, 'How do nurses learn through experience in clinical practice?' There were four sub-questions:

1. What experiences in practice are significant for nurses with regard to learning practical knowledge?
2. What meanings are embedded in these experiences?
3. What features in the context of the experiences influence nurses' subsequent practice?
4. What is the nature of learning in these experiences?

As the field work began new understandings were gained and these specific questions quickly became too limiting as I found the notion of experience to be less clear-cut than I had taken it to be. Rather than replacing these questions with other specific questions, they were kept in abeyance. As the research progressed, I kept the two principles of the nurse-in-context and 'keeping close' to experience, at the forefront of my mind and continued to explore how meaning, learning and knowledge were revealed in the nurses' experiences and practices.

As excellent, experienced nurses were selected to participate in the study, I felt that I could not simply focus generally on learning through experience, so the general question was re-orientated early in the period of field work to: 'How do nurses develop expertise in clinical nursing practice?' Some time later, when I was well into the analysis, I was beginning to understand that, in addition to everyday experience, I was looking at nursing practices and the process of practising expertly. Everyday experiences provided a window onto nursing practices, and by examining how nurses experience practice on a moment-by-moment, day-by-day basis, another window was opened, this one onto the process of practice. A question, 'How do nurses practise expertly?', was added. It must be said that although the questions served to focus aspects of the study, the overall goal remained intact: namely, to explore the nature of everyday experience and its contribution to the development of clinical expertise.

THE NURSES AND THEIR SETTING

The study was undertaken in a large Scottish city. Following contact with the Health Board's Chief Area Nursing Officer, an initial exploratory meeting was held with the Area Nursing Officer responsible for research. She contacted the Directors of Nursing Services of two acute care hospitals and secured permission for me to contact them. Both hospitals were multi-specialty, university-affiliated hospitals involved in research and the education of medical, nursing and paramedical personnel. One hospital was large (over 900 beds); the other smaller (over 400 beds).

Initially, I asked for 'qualified nurses who are acknowledged to be experts in surgical nursing'. I specifically wished to study nurses in adult 'general' surgical nursing units for the following reasons.

I am most familiar with surgical nursing of adult patients. My clinical experience is not extensive. Prior to the study, while working in nursing administration, I maintained a connection with a surgical ward, occasionally participating in patient care and assisting with the development of primary nursing.

Nurses are often expected to gain 'basic experience' in general surgery. Nurses working in this area are not considered to be specialists; there are no post-basic courses offered in general surgical nursing. For the most part, nurses in these areas develop their particular nursing knowledge through self-study and practical experience. For the purpose of observation, the 'pace' of these wards is often more rapid than the other area with which I am familiar, Geriatrics. I expected that there would be more opportunities to observe nurses in a broader range of practice in surgery.

Prior to my discussions with the Directors of Nursing Services I had not determined what would count as 'general' surgical nursing units, except to exclude intensive therapy units.

At my initial meetings with them, the Directors of Nursing Services expressed interest in the study and a willingness to participate. We discussed the term 'expert', noting how unfamiliar it was in the Scottish nursing context and agreed that it would be more comfortable to speak of 'excellent, experienced' nurses, a term I used for the remainder of the study.

The nurses

Nurses were selected by the Directors of Nursing Services using the following criteria:

1. Employed in nursing clinical practice for at least 5 years.
2. Currently engaged in direct patient care in a surgical nursing setting.
3. Identified by colleagues as highly skilled clinical practice nurses.
4. Employed full-time in nursing.
5. Registered general nurses.

These criteria were used by Benner (1984) and others (Olsen 1985, Crabtree & Jorgenson 1986, Benner & Tanner 1987) to identify expert nurses.

In Benner's (1984) study, the expert nurses were selected by staff development directors in consultation with head nurses and peers. Crabtree & Jorgenson (1986) selected a random sample from eligible nurses identified through responses to a mailed questionnaire. Several years ago, Hyslop (1987) expressed concern regarding the use of peer nomination as a means of selecting expert nurses in Scotland. In his study of expert decision-making on pressure sores, he selected expert nurses through self-report and an assessment test, noting that nurses do not work together enough to allow them to nominate their peers as experts.

In the initial discussions with the Directors of Nursing Services, I stressed that numbers were unimportant; my main concerns were that the nurses were excellent, experienced surgical nurses and that they would be willing to participate in this in-depth study. Both Directors said that nurses who met the criteria immediately came to mind. Following the meeting, in consultation with their senior nursing officers for the surgical areas, the Directors selected nurses for participation in the study. Seven nurses were identified at the larger hospital, and three at the smaller one. One Director said that she and her colleague had separately identified nurses and had found that in six of seven cases they were the same. Originally I wanted to study 15 nurses, but found that there was more than ample material generated in the study of 10.

The nurses selected were eight ward sisters and two staff nurses. They are referred to in the study by pseudonyms. At the time of the study, nine of the nurses worked full-time; one of the staff nurses, though part-time, had worked for many years on one ward and conducted a weekly outpatient clinic. The second staff nurse was an acting ward sister during part of the study, and was promoted to ward sister following the period of field work. Both staff nurses had responsibilities which would normally be undertaken by a ward sister. For this reason, I have called all of the nurses 'Ward Sisters' for the purposes of the study. Where the nurse's role as a staff nurse was pertinent to the analysis, it has been mentioned.

In the text, the nurses are usually referred to by their title and surname and this is how they are referred to in the course of their workday. On only a few occasions did I hear co-workers use the nurses' first names.

All of the Ward Sisters have extensive experiences in nursing. In the spring of 1988, at the completion of the field work, all the Sisters had been qualified nurses for between six and 33 years. Five Sisters had between six and 12 years of experience, the remainder had between 24 and 33 years of experience. Most of their experience had been in surgical nursing and they had been in their current posts for between 2.5 and 12 years, the mean being 6.5 years. The Sisters are experienced, clinically qualified nurses. By and large, the nurses in the study continued their education by taking clinical courses and study opportunities which related to their clinical work.

All of the British-born Sisters qualified as registered general nurses (RGN or SRN); two trained initially in England, eight in Scotland. One initially trained as a Registered Orthopaedic Nurse. Another qualified as a district nurse as part of her basic nursing after studying nursing initially at a university and taking a bachelor's degree. At the time of the study, one nurse was studying part-time for a social sciences degree.

Following registration, several of the nurses acquired additional qualifications: one became a Registered Sick Children's Nurse; two trained as midwives. Three took the year-long Intensive Care course, one took an Ear, Nose and Throat course, one took an Oncology Nursing course, another an Enterostomal Therapy course. Two have taken a 6-week Care of the Dying course, one a Family Planning course and three a health education short course. The eight sisters had taken at least one Introduction to Management course. All, save for one part-time staff nurse, had attended a variety of study days. At the time of the study, the continuing education opportunity provided by the hospital for the part-time nurse had consisted of a fire lecture.

In these hospitals, as in many others on both sides of the Atlantic, it is not unusual for certain nurses to be 'volunteered', or encouraged to participate in research studies or developmental projects. Often these nurses are amongst the informal leaders in the organization who can be counted on to test system changes fairly or to lead organizational developments. It is notable that during the period of field work and afterwards, sisters in the study were involved in, among other projects: testing a new medication administration system, a work analysis programme, and leading the development of nursing standards. Several of the wards were frequently used by the Colleges of Nursing for students or staff who needed extra assessment or developmental work.

Not all of the Sisters were enthusiastic volunteers. Two in particular were reluctant to participate. I gave them the opportunity to decline, but admittedly, given the process of selection, it was difficult for them to opt out of the study[1]. Therefore, with all of the Sisters, and with them in particular, I made every effort to match the field work schedule and my way of working to their needs. On a number of previous occasions, I had created a cooperative work situation with people who were initially reluctant or actually hostile. With some of the Sisters in particular, I drew on all of this developmental experience and stretched my skills. I was especially sensitive to being in an unfamiliar cultural and social situation. My success can perhaps be judged by the fact that all of the Sisters participated fully and openly throughout the duration of the study; none of them was stinting in their involvement.

The wards

Although nurses on general surgical wards were requested, it is perhaps instructive of the state of specialization in surgical nursing that only two of the 10 wards are actually general surgical wards. The wards in the study were as follows:

- ear, nose and throat
- general surgery
- gynaecology
- orthopaedic trauma
- thoracic surgery
- urology
- vascular surgery.

The wards ranged in size from 20 to 36 beds. Three of the larger wards were mixed-sex wards, four were male wards and three held female patients only. Six wards were Nightingale-style; four were comprised of rooms for smaller numbers of patients. All wards undertook a mix of in-patient surgery and same-day surgery.

FIELD WORK

Access to the two hospitals was negotiated in June and July 1987. The field work began in August 1987 and continued until June 1988. Field work consisted of two periods of observation and three interviews with each Sister. In addition, a group interview was held. From August to November 1987, I 'shadowed' each Sister for 5 days and conducted the first interview shortly thereafter. Between December 1987 and February 1988, I interviewed each Sister a second time. Between March and June 1988, I shadowed the Sisters again for 2 days and conducted the third interview in the afternoon of the third day. The group interview was held with seven Sisters in mid-June 1988.

Participant observation: shadowing the sisters

It was originally intended that the interviews would provide the main source of material for analysis and the period of participant observation would provide me with a sense of the context, and therefore enable a better interpretation of the interview material. During the first day of observation it became apparent to me that many practices were effective because of the Sisters' particular movements, their use of personal space, timing, pacing and voice intonations. I was picking up 'the kinesic dimension of professional performance' (Dingwall 1976), i.e. the Sisters' comportment. I realized at the time that this dimension was critical to the Sisters' effectiveness in practice yet would not be talked about in the interview situation as it was so taken for granted. Thus, I approached the participant observation in such a way that I could gain the maximum amount in the limited time I had with each Sister.

The literature on participant observation stresses the need to spend time immersing oneself in the situation in order to understand the 'matrix of meanings' of those studied (Emerson 1987). As a nurse, I already had access to many of the meanings and much of the professional knowledge. On the one hand, my prior knowledge was critical as I attempted to follow what each Sister was doing in the course of her clinical practice. On the other hand, I was unfamiliar with the Scottish nursing practice context and particularities of treatment modalities as my nursing experience had taken place entirely in Canada.

Common problems for the participant observer, such as when to be in the field, where to stand and what to observe, were somewhat simplified for me. Quite literally, I shadowed the Sisters throughout the course of their workday for 5 consecutive shifts in the first phase of the field work, and two consecutive shifts in the second. The period of 5 days was chosen to give me a chance to be with each Sister within a 3-month period. There were considerable scheduling difficulties; any longer than 5 days would have been impossible to implement within that time. Although the Sisters often work for longer periods, 5 days allowed me to capture a sense of their experience of a working week. For two Sisters, it was impossible to schedule 5 days, so I was with them for 4 days apiece. I was with each Sister for her entire shift (which often lasted 9 hours); the part-time Sister worked 4 hours each day. Early and late shifts, weekdays and weekends were included. In the first phase of the field work, I observed the Sisters for a total of 360 hours.

In the third phase of the field work, my intent was to observe the Sister for a sufficient period of time to become familiar again with her practice and to provide the basis for discussion. I was with all but one of the Sisters for two consecutive shifts, for a total observation time of 128 hours. The interview was held in the afternoon of the second shift. As one of the Sisters was 'acting up' as the nursing officer at the time, I did not observe her in practice. I interviewed her, however, about practices which I had previously observed.

In the hospital wards, I wore nurses' shoes, a white laboratory coat over street clothes, and a badge identifying me as 'Martha MacLeod RN, Nursing Research Student, University of Edinburgh'. Each Sister had a different way of introducing me on the ward. I was usually introduced to the doctors and nursing staff as a 'Nursing researcher who is studying me and how I work. She will be with us for the week'. All of the Sisters were aware that I am registered to practice as a general nurse in the United Kingdom. Some mentioned the fact in their introductions to staff. To the longer-term patients I was introduced as 'Martha MacLeod, a Canadian nurse who is doing research'; I was often not introduced to patients who were on the ward for a short period of time.

The Sisters included me in virtually all their activities. I was not included in two 'difficult' student assessments, and on one occasion at medical rounds, the consultant and the Sister went to look at a woman's anal cyst, leaving the registrars, residents and me in the hallway. On all other occasions, including giving relatives news of a patient's death, meeting with a staff nurse for the first time and being 'behind the curtains', I was there. The Sisters did not attend administrative meetings while I was with them, so I did not observe that aspect of their work. My participation in care was limited, but I helped to lift and turn patients, make beds, tidy work areas and answer the telephone. When shadowing one of the staff nurses, the patient assignment was done with an acknowledgement that I would be available to help in a limited way with the bathing, lifting and turning. At all times, my participation in care was at the Sister's request and happened with her.

When I shadowed the Sisters, I stood where I could see their faces and the patients' faces and hear their conversations. I was part of the group receiving the ward reports, and at doctors' rounds stood where I could see and hear the Sisters' interactions. I wear a hearing aid that enables me to hear 'normally'; however, I am particularly attentive to faces, and I made sure that I stood where that was possible. During the field work, my main difficulty was catching what the consultants said during rounds.

My attention during participant observation was focused on a Sister's practices: what she was attending to, what she was doing and how what she was doing fitted with and formed the situation. I watched and listened for the responses of others to the Sister's actions. I continually had to try to make sense of what was going on. Just as Atkinson (1984) found he learned about medicine while studying medical students, I found that I was learning about each of the clinical specialties so I could understand what the Sisters were doing. The first day was particularly difficult as I had to become familiar with the new pace, people, concerns and language of the ward. After the first day, in which I mostly listened and watched, I often asked the Sisters what they saw, or what they were thinking. They were used to having students around and frequently, spontaneously explained what they were doing, why they were doing it and what they were going to do next. This was invaluable.

My presence was, by all accounts, well accepted. I seemed to be perceived by patients and staff, not so much as an intruder, but more as 'an extension' of the Sisters for the time I was with them (Kratz 1975). The Sisters said that they found me comfortable to have around. They were surprised at this, as most had not looked forward to being so closely observed. My age and previous administrative position did not seem to influence the field work negatively. I am older than half of the Sisters. They related to me as a Canadian student, a researcher and a nurse. While I recognize the limitations of my insights into the Sisters' world of practice afforded by such a short period of participant observation, their openness enabled me to get the most out of that time.

I took notes in a small notebook throughout the shift. As many others are taking notes in hand-over reports, my note-taking was not obtrusive then or during rounds. I often jotted down reminders and phrases while the Sister was on the telephone, writing in the kardex, or doing some paperwork herself. One Sister said that she often forgot I was there except when my pen came out. After that, I tried to make my note-taking even more unobtrusive. On the other hand, two Sisters asked me to take a couple of reminder notes for them, and another used the times I had written down to confirm her understanding of a situation. Following each day of participant observation, I created field notes on the computer from my jottings. This was difficult to maintain given the work schedule, but usually they were completed within 2 days, and in all cases the field notes from my time with one Sister were completed before shadowing the next.

The interviews

Each Sister was interviewed three times, with 3 months between each interview. The interviews were held in the Sister's room or another office on the ward, during her regular working hours. Each interview lasted between 35 minutes and 2 hours; the average was 80 minutes. The later interviews, without exception, lasted longer than the first interviews. The interviews were tape recorded and the recordings transcribed verbatim.

Before the beginning of the field work, two practice interviews were held with two undergraduate nursing students. The interview format for my first interview with the Sisters was used. These practice interviews helped me to get used to the tape recorder and alerted me to some abruptness in my interviewing technique, which I subsequently modified.

The interviews could be characterized as reflexive interviews (Hammersley & Atkinson 1983). There was an underlying structure and agenda which I determined, but the direction in which the interview developed was influenced by, amongst other things, the experiences related by the Sisters, our ease with each other and the Sisters' current work concerns. I approached each interview with a goal in mind, an opening question, areas to discuss and probes. The questions and probes are detailed in MacLeod (1990). I followed Bogdan & Taylor's (1975 p 108) maxim that what is ultimately important in a qualitative interview, is a clear frame of reference. The interviews were much like those described by Tough (1982): intensive, probing, medium-paced (almost leisurely at times), and in-depth.

In the first interview, the Sisters were asked to describe experiences in their practice, for example, a situation in which they made a difference to a patient, a situation that went unusually well or one that was very ordinary and typical. The questions and probes were taken from Benner (1984). Unlike Benner's (1984) and Crabtree & Jorgenson's (1986) studies, I did not provide an outline of the kind of description I was interested in prior to the interviews. Only one of the Sisters asked me before the interview what kinds of questions I would be asking, and when I told her, came prepared with some 'stories' [her word] to tell me. At the beginning of the interview, the Sisters did not find it easy to tell me about their own experiences, but once they had related one, they readily told me about other experiences with memorable patients. Two nurses in particular talked about what they normally did in situations; I found myself continually asking them for specific examples, which they willingly provided. The forms of the experiences told in the interviews are discussed in relation to the nature of experience in Chapter 4.

As many of the experiences and memorable patients discussed in the first interview pertained to situations early in the Sisters' careers, my goal for the second interview was to hear about more recent experiences, and for the Sisters to make links, when they could, between these and earlier or subsequent experiences. In this interview, the Sisters gave me specifics without my having to probe; they no longer asked if they were 'going on' or were 'off on a tangent'. Two or three of the Sisters also told me about situations of which they had thought at the time, 'Martha would be interested in this'. These situations were ones in which a simple nursing action had made a difference to a patient.

The first and second interviews elicited few very recent experiences and there were considerable areas of their practice which the Sisters did not talk about at all. Therefore, I began the third interview by asking the Sisters to tell me about the last 2 days. I then moved on to commenting on two or three of their practices which I had observed, and asked them if they remembered when they did not do them as well. The con-

centration in this interview was more on their learning and influences on that learning. In this interview, I also asked about their education and work experience.

The interviews took place at the Sisters' convenience, usually in their room on the ward. We were seldom interrupted. The interviews were recorded by a small hand-held tape recorder placed between us. None of the Sisters particularly liked being recorded and one person strongly voiced her concerns, but nevertheless agreed to be taped. This same person commented at the beginning of the third interview that she felt crowded by where I had sat in the second interview, so I moved to where it was comfortable for her. At the same time as expressing her dislike of interviews, she commented on how easy it was for her to have me shadow her.

To conclude the field work, I held a 1.5-hour group interview with seven of the 10 Sisters, exploring themes I found amongst them all. One Sister came in from holidays for the interview; staffing difficulties prevented two from attending and one was out of the country. They commented later on how nice it was to get together.

I added my comments about the interview to the tape following each interview; they were transcribed along with the interviews. All of the interviews were transcribed verbatim in the first instance by an assistant. I listened to all the tapes, checked the transcription and ensured all were complete. Often discussed amongst researchers, but seldom included in research reports, is the question about the necessity for a complete transcription, including the normal grunts, repetitions and other flotsam of normal speech. These were included in the transcriptions because they are a normal part of language, and can point towards the emotional content, the ease of expression and the character of the experience being recounted. However, even with a complete transcription of an oral conversation, the language is, of necessity, transformed. The written artifact can never capture all of the vividness, the pacing and the non-verbal aspects of the conversation.

The interviews have been edited for the sake of clarity. In making these editorial changes the intention has been to achieve 'fidelity to the participants' meaning' (Weber 1986). The changes have been made with the encouragement of the Sisters. Indeed, upon reading the first drafts of the interpretation, they requested changes in their dialect or use of colloquialisms to make them 'sound more professional'. In most instances, these changes were made with the recognition that there are different 'forms of talk'. 'Public talk' is often more coherently presented than the 'private talk' which is captured in tape recordings of conversations, albeit interview conversations (S Tilley, personal communication, 1990).

A HERMENEUTIC INTERPRETATION

In this study, the interview transcripts and field notes were treated as text, or text analogues and a hermeneutic interpretation was carried out with them. Hermeneutics derives from a reference to Hermes, the Greek messenger god, who had to understand and interpret a multiplicity of messages, languages and meanings of the various gods, so that he could translate and convey their meaning to mortals. Hermeneutics is an 'attempt to make clear, to make sense of an object of study' (Taylor 1971). Originally, hermeneutic interpretations were only undertaken on written texts but Ricoeur (1979) successfully made the case for the applicability of hermeneutic interpretation to both action and speech. Ricoeur argued that language in discourse, both written and spoken, can be fixed and thus become the subject of hermeneutic interpretation. This is no less so for meaningful action which can be described. When discourse and action are inscribed into texts and text analogues, they become distanced from the writer, speaker or actor. 'The author's intention and the meaning of the text cease to coincide' (Ricoeur 1979). They are thus differently placed in the intersubjective realm. The world and situation of the discourse can then be addressed more readily.

The process of hermeneutic interpretation as proposed here is underpinned by the following principles:

The researcher enters into dialogue with the text (Gadamer 1975). The interview, a work of discourse, tells a story about a particular topic or issue (Honey 1987). In this case, the story is about nursing experience. The statements within the story, both those of the Sisters and mine, could be considered responses to questions. As Gadamer (1981 p 106) says, to get hold of the statement of the text is to get hold of the question to which the statement is an answer. To put it another way:

'Interpretation is a response to questions put not solely by the interpreting subject to an object, the text ... It is a response to questions raised by the subject matter of the text.' (Llewelyn 1985 p 115).

Thus, the interpreter needs to attend to what the text is saying, and to the question to which it is responding. 'A good interpreter must be a good listener' (Llewelyn 1985 p 111).

Unlike other forms of phenomenology (Omery 1983, Giorgi 1975, 1985), in hermeneutic phenomenology the researcher does not 'bracket' his or her presuppositions, reduce the phenomena and stand outside the text. Rather than being disengaged, the researcher is reflective but engaged within the situation (Packer 1985). The process of interpretation stemming from engagement with the situation may be characterized by Gadamer's (1975) notion of a 'fusion of horizons'. Our horizon, according to Gadamer, is our range of vision which includes everything that can be seen from a particular vantage point. The horizon of the present is constituted, as mentioned in a previous section, by our background, or pre-understandings. As they are not separate from us, they are impossible to see beyond. However, through engagement and dialogue, the horizons of the present can be transcended. It could be said that our horizon is something that moves with us as we encounter the world. Gadamer makes the point that interpretation is a process imbued with time:

In fact the horizon of the present is being continually formed, in that we have continually to test all our prejudices. An important part of this testing is the encounter with the past and the understanding of the tradition from which we come. Hence the horizon of the present cannot be formed without the past. There is no more an isolated horizon of the present than there are historical horizons. Understanding, rather, is always the fusion of these horizons which we imagine to exist by themselves. (Gadamer 1975 p 273)

The researcher as interpreter comes into the act of interpretation with a set of personal pre-conceptions or prejudices and a theoretical lens (Kuhn 1977). Through the process of interpretation, these become more clearly articulated in relation to the text. Rather than trying to get free of 'researcher bias', the researcher attempts to recognize her influence on the interpretation while attempting to fully hear the voice of the text.

Thus it can be argued that the meaning of an action or text (or text analogue) does not rest only in the writer, actor or speaker, nor in the interpreter alone, but is constituted in both.

The process is not linear. It is characterized by the hermeneutic circle. Central to the notion of the hermeneutic circle is the interplay of the parts and the whole. To understand the whole, the parts are understood, part by part, so that a progressively more complete awareness of the whole is grasped. The comprehension of each part, however, is enriched by the understanding of the overall whole. In this way, the hermeneutic circle gives a direction for the method of interpretation to be used by the researcher. Understanding happens as a whole and not merely as the addition of discrete elements. The hermeneutic circle has implications for the form of analysis. That is, the analysis cannot be linear, nor can it consist of categorizing the text into discrete elements and compiling them into broader categories or composites. The data are not 'distilled' into its essence. Instead, coming to understanding is a rather messy process of moving reflexively between parts and the whole, beyond the parts and the whole and back again.

The process of analysis is systematic, a 'dialectic of guessing and validation' (Ricoeur 1979). Throughout the process of interpretation, the horizon of understanding is tested and reformed through the process of dialogue with the text. As a part of this process of guessing and validation, the researcher is constantly making comparisons amongst instances in the text (cf. Glaser & Strauss 1967, Glaser 1978) and amongst the evolving themes and their interplay with the text. **The goal is not to understand the text, but to understand something in front of it — the human project (Heidegger 1962, Rabinow & Sullivan 1979).** The interpretation which is sought is a new creation, a synthesis of the horizons of both the text and the interpreter. The interpretation does not lie underneath, nor behind the text, but rather in-between the text and the interpreter. The interpretation sought in this study is not the Sisters' interpretation of their own situation, nor is it merely my interpretation. Instead, I am aiming at an interpretation which brings to light what the Sisters already understand about their experience and practices, but bringing them to light in new way, in a new interpretation, one beyond their own.

Universals or theories are not identified through this process, rather human context and world are explicated (Rabinow & Sullivan 1979). The interpretation discloses the complexities and interrelatedness of meanings in context. Within the perspective of hermeneutic phenomenology one can never be clear of the context, if for no other reason than that language embodies the cultural world within which the researcher and research participants live (Taylor 1971). Thus, context-free theories would provide too skeletal a view of the Sisters' experience and practices.

The second characteristic of the hermeneutic circle also figures here. Within hermeneutic interpretation, there is never a final or absolute interpretation.

We cannot escape an ultimate appeal to a common understanding of the expressions, of the 'language' involved ... What we are trying to establish is a certain reading of text or expressions, and what we appeal to as our grounds for this reading can only be other readings. (Taylor 1971 p 6)

It is not an arbitrary interpretation which is sought, but one which best makes sense in this place and time. As Strong (1979 p 250) states, 'The best we can hope for in this world, even if we study practical reasoning, is a plausible story'. I would argue that for a broader credibility, the interpretation in this study must also make theoretical sense (Silverman 1989). Having said that, it is most important that the interpretation is recognizable by the Sisters and others who are familiar with situations such as theirs.

Interpreting the interview transcripts and field notes

The field notes were written and the interview audiotapes transcribed. The material for all of the nurses totalled 2500 pages of text, about 250 pages per Sister. A major challenge was to find a way to keep a sense of the whole, whilst analysing parts. In comparison to Knafl & Webster (1988), who suggest that data management activities are undertaken merely to prepare data for analysis, I would argue that the management of data in itself is part of the analytical and interpretative process. This is particularly so when the aim is not to reduce the data to pieces and subsequently reassemble them, but rather to come to an ever richer understanding of the parts and the whole.

The interview transcripts and field notes were assembled for each Sister. I worked on a paper copy with a wide right hand margin. My original intention was to begin by reading the material as a whole for all the Sisters as Diekelmann et al (1989) suggest. This proved to be too daunting a task, so I decided to work with the material for one Sister at a time. In the first instance, I read the material as a whole without taking notes. I then took each day of field notes and each interview. I began with the field notes, in order to get the context of work and took the interviews in the order: 3, 1, 2.

Keeping the two principles, the nurse-in-context and 'keeping close' to experience, in mind, I asked these questions as I went through the text:

- What is going on here?
- What is the nature of experience?
- What is knowing in this situation and how does it show up?
- What learning is here? How does it happen?
- What is the nature of the situation?
- What is the temporal nature of the experience?
- What does this particular situation/aspects of the situation link to — and how do they link?

I was unable to identify a firm 'unit of analysis' or 'meaning unit' (Giorgi 1985). Benner (1984), Diekelmann (1989) and others used the paradigm case as the unit of analysis; however, the experiences in these study interviews did not all fall into the form of paradigm cases and exemplars. Brykczynski's (1985) study used discrete nurse-patient encounters as units of analysis, in addition to paradigm cases. However, the field notes in this study took a different form, following the variety, complexity and discontinuity of the Sisters' work.

Trying to identify a unit of analysis, however, was useful because I was pushed into considering the form of experiences. When an 'experience' could not be readily identified, I asked myself, What is this then? In addition to considering the content of the interviews, I examined the turns in the conversations — where they came from, what seemed to be happening and where the turn led. Reading the field notes, I asked: What makes up an experience? Whose experience is it — mine or the Sisters'? I explored the character of experience around a single patient, situation or group of patients over a period of days in the field notes, between interviews and between field notes and interviews.

During this process, I highlighted what stood out, wrote brief margin notes and then went through the notes and text again, making further notes on separate sheets under the four headings of Experience, Knowledge, Learning and Flavour, and linking them to instances in the text. After completing these notes for all of the material for one Sister, I read them through and identified ideas or questions, writing them on file cards. These ideas were much like overlapping, amorphous categories with a quote attached, and/or thoughts which they provoked. I considered them to be worth exploring further. For example, cards were created with the titles, 'little things, helping, doctor-nurse relationship, safety net, wounds, comfort, staffing, noticing'. For each Sister, I created a new set of cards and labels. I did not seek to fit the ideas into discrete categories, but during this process, I was identifying where ideas/issues (e.g. authority) showed up and where they did not, and how they were different between Sisters and among experiences. Throughout this process, there was a continual interplay between the parts and the whole, within an interview or day of field notes, and between the parts and whole of material for each Sister.

For each Sister, I made a card 'Flavour' with quotes and situations which particularly stood out, and another card, 'Knowledge', in which I cited examples in relation to Benner's (1984) domains. I did not attempt to bring out all of the possibilities in the text: the material is so rich I would still be analysing it. Instead, I worked with each Sister's material until I thought I knew it well, and had grasped as much as possible in it. This process took three 40-hour weeks for the first Sister's material, two weeks for the second, four for the third, and between one and two weeks for each of the other Sisters' material.

As part of this process, colleagues read excerpts from the text and we compared analyses. It was particularly useful on two counts: for helping me to be more clear about my prejudices, and for looking at the text from more than one angle.

The next stage was to review the cards and notes which I had made for myself. (These were much like Glaser's (1978) theoretical memos.) I made piles of cards with similar ideas and looked for patterns and areas of dissimilarity within and among them. I also looked at how they fitted with Experience, Knowledge and Learning. I was trying to get a sense of the whole for all of the nurses and how the parts fitted in. At this stage, I was identifying loose themes (e.g. knowing the patient). I discussed these with colleagues and with two of the Sisters who said that they made sense to them.

I began writing at this point, creating a description of each Sister's practice. This description highlighted a lack of pattern in the material and the fact that I had not adequately grasped the whole. I then spent three weeks in front of a blackboard with the material, searching for patterns. A number of themes emerged, such as: nursing practice – experience with individuals; nursing practice – experience with groups; the process of practising; the process of learning through experience. These themes and central links amongst the themes

were further developed through writing several drafts of the chapters.

A great deal of the interpretation and understanding has occurred through writing and re-writing. As Van Manen (1984 p 68) says, 'To write phenomenologically is the untiring effort to author a sensitive grasp of being itself . . . ' I have found that I have needed to work at developing a style of writing which conveys the nature of everyday experience.

To write, to work at style, is to exercise an interpretative tact, which in the sense of style produces the thinking/writing body of text . . . But we should not confuse style with mere technique or method; rather, style shows and reflects what the author is capable of seeing and showing in the way that he or she is oriented to the world and to language. (Van Manen 1989 p 242)

The interpretation which is presented here has developed and changed through the various drafts of this study.

The Sisters were involved at several points in the development of the interpretation. In June 1989, 1 year after I had left the field, I met with six of the Sisters to present a paper to them '"He's better in himself": nurses' knowledge of the patient recovering from surgery'. Their response was warm. One Sister said, 'What you say makes what we do sound important!' She paused and continued, 'Of course it is, but I mean, it's just what we do'. Another Sister, who had read the first draft of one chapter, said about it, 'It is easy to read and riveting. The only down side is that the not so nice aspects of our practice aren't shown'. Over the next five months all of the Sisters read all of the analysis chapters in first draft. Overall, they agreed with the interpretations and made specific corrections, such as the names of medications and the sequence of a procedure. One Sister said that she had taken the section, 'Making the ward work', to her husband and said to him, 'Read this. This is what I do!' Another Sister wrote: 'Many things which you have mentioned in your paper have helped me understand the situation more . . . '.

Late in 1989, I presented a paper, 'Attuned to experience: how nurses practise expertly', to the Sisters before giving it elsewhere. They pointed out some unclear wording but supported the interpretation. A spirited discussion about the importance of caring and the nature of expertise followed.

ISSUES OF ETHICS AND RIGOUR

Confidentiality has been perhaps the most difficult ethical issue in this research. At the outset, I promised confidentiality to the Sisters. The names used throughout are pseudonyms; however, it is quite possible that within their milieux they could be identified. I raised this issue of confidentiality with them as soon as it became apparent to me that I could not avoid the potential of disclosure if the context were to remain intact. We discussed this at length and the Sisters have agreed with the approach I have taken. As one wrote after reading the draft chapters, 'It is unfortunate that the Sisters concerned can be identified by their specialties but I cannot see how you can avoid this as it is necessary to the context of the paper'. The move to name all of the nurses, including the two staff nurses, 'Sister' may lessen the potential of their identification. At no point have the Sisters asked that a situation be omitted. Only minor modifications have been requested. For example, one Sister requested that reference to a specialty be removed from an example in which she was talking about previous experiences as she felt another person might be identifiable.

The Sisters have been consistently supportive of my creating an open and balanced interpretation of their practice and experience. The apparent lack of 'negative' instances of practice in the preceding chapters is not an oversight. It occurs for two reasons. Although I was not out to evaluate practice, interpreting the quality of situations is an unavoidable part of understanding them. When observing, you see the effect of actions as well as the actions themselves.

The examples provided in the book are representative of the Sisters' practice. They described many days that I was with them as typical days. I did not observe instances of 'poor' practice. That is not to say that the Sisters

did not think they could have handled situations better. There were also instances in which I could have suggested an alternate approach, but their approaches made sense in the situation. The Sister who made the comment about the lack of negative instances said she was thinking of a time when she did not handle well the timing of attending to relatives of a patient who had died. My understanding of the situation was tempered by the realization of the tremendous number of other details she was attending to at the same time in an extraordinarily difficult situation. I marvelled that she timed it as well as she did.

The second reason for a 'positive' description is the perspective offered by hermeneutic phenomenology. The approach leads to focusing on what is there in language and practices, not on what is lacking. It does not provide a deficit view (Benner 1985).

Throughout this discussion, I have attempted to highlight the points of decision, so readers may examine them. Although I would argue that reliability in the usual sense is not possible because of the contextual nature of the research and the individuality of the researcher, there is a need to address the reliability of the interpretation (Silverman 1989). The openness and details in this appendix are an attempt to establish the trustworthiness of my interpretation. A credible, robust interpretation has been sought through such means as: creating a rich source of material for interpretation from participant observation, multiple interviews with individual participants and one group interview; undertaking the interpretation in multiple stages; testing out the interpretation with the participants and colleagues; undertaking a style of research which is within the capacity and skills of the researcher. The fruits of these efforts are revealed in the consistency, depth and coherence of the account in the preceding chapters.

Notes

[1] At the time of the study, a consent form for staff's participation in research was not required by the Health Board or either hospital. In lieu of a consent form, I sent a letter to each participant, confirming my involvement and her participation.

References

Abel P, Kerr S, Urquhart J, Ilsley R 1986 Nursing line management in Scotland. Scottish Health Service Studies no 46. Scottish Home and Health Department, Edinburgh

Adam E 1987 Nursing theory: what it is and what it is not. Nursing Papers: Perspectives in Nursing 19(2): 5–14

Akin G 1991a Varieties of managerial learning. Journal of Health Administration Education 11(2): 167–177

Akin G 1991b Commentary. Journal of Health Administration Education 11(2): 179–185

Alexander M 1980 Nurse education: an experiment in integration of theory and practice in nursing. PhD thesis, University of Edinburgh

Alexander M F, Fawcett J N, Runciman P J (eds) 1994 Nursing practice hospital and home — the adult. Churchill Livingstone, Edinburgh

Allen D G, Bowers B, Diekelmann N 1989 Writing to learn: a reconceptualization of thinking and writing in the nursing curriculum. Journal of Nursing Education 28(1): 6–11

Allen H O 1982 The ward sister: role and preparation. Baillière Tindall, London

Altschul A T 1979 Commitment to nursing. Journal of Advanced Nursing 4: 123–135

Argyris C, Schön D 1974 Theory in practice. Jossey-Bass, San Francisco

Argyris C 1993 Knowledge for action: a guide to overcoming barriers to organizational change. Jossey-Bass, San Francisco

Atkinson P 1981 The clinical experience: the construction and reconstruction of medical reality. Gower, Aldershott

Atkinson P 1984 Wards and deeds: taking knowledge and control seriously. In: Burgess R G (ed) The research process in educational settings: 10 case studies. The Falmer Press, London

Attridge C, Callahan M 1989 Women in women's work: nurses, stress and power. Recent Advances in Nursing 25: 41–69

Auld M G 1988 Nursing services 1977–1987. Health Bulletin 46(2): 76–86

Baker C A 1989 Recovery: a phenomenon extending beyond discharge. Scholarly Inquiry for Nursing Practice: An International Journal 3(3): 181–194

Bandura A 1977 Social learning theory. Prentice-Hall, Englewood Cliffs, New Jersey

Barker P 1989 Rules of engagement. Nursing Times 85(15): 58–60

Beck C T 1994 Phenomenology: its use in nursing research. International Journal of Nursing Studies 31(6): 499–510

Beckstrand J 1978 The notion of a practice theory and the relationship of scientific and ethical knowledge to practice. Research in Nursing and Health 1(3): 131–136

Bellezza F 1986 Mental cues and verbal reports in learning. In: Bower G H (ed) The psychology of learning and motivation: advances in research and theory, vol 2. Academic Press, New York

Bendall E 1973 The relationship between recall and application of learning in trainee nurses. PhD thesis, University of London

Bendall E 1975 So you passed, Nurse. An exploration of some of the assumptions on which written examinations are based. Royal College of Nursing, London

Benner P 1982 Issues in competency-based testing. Nursing Outlook (May): 303–309

Benner P 1983 Uncovering the knowledge embedded in clinical practice. Image: The Journal of Nursing Scholarship 15(2): 36–41

Benner P 1984 From novice to expert: excellence and power in clinical nursing practice. Addison-Wesley, Menlo Park, California

Benner P 1985 Quality of life: a phenomenological perspective on explanation, prediction and understanding in nursing science. Advances in Nursing Science 81: 1–14

Benner P 1987 A dialogue with excellence. American Journal of Nursing (September): 1170–1172

Benner P 1988 Nursing as a caring profession. Paper presented at the American Academy of Nursing, 16–18 October, Kansas City, Missouri

Benner P 1991 The role of experience, narrative, and community in skilled ethical comportment. Advances in Nursing Science 14(2): 1–21

Benner P (ed) 1994 Interpretative phenomenology: embodiment, caring and ethics in health and illness. Sage, London

Benner P, Tanner C 1987 How expert nurses use intuition. American Journal of Nursing (January): 23–31

Benner P, Tanner C, Chesla C 1992 From beginner to expert: gaining a differentiated clinical world in critical care nursing. Advances in Nursing Science 14(3): 13–28

Benner P, Wrubel J 1982 Skilled clinical knowledge: the value of perceptual awareness. Nurse Educator (May-June): 11–17

Benner P, Wrubel J 1989 The primacy of caring: stress and coping in health and illness. Addison-Wesley, Menlo Park, California

Bereiter C, Scardamalia M 1986 Educational relevance of the study of expertise. Interchange 172: 10–24

Berger P, Luckmann T 1967 The social construction of reality. Penguin, Harmondsworth

Bergman R, Stockler R A, Shavit N, Sharon R, Feinberg D, Danon A 1981 Role, selection and preparation of unit head nurses — III. International Journal of Nursing Studies 18(4): 237–250

Bigge M L 1982 Learning theories for teachers, 4th edn. Harper & Row, New York

Blumer H 1969 Symbolic interactionism. Prentice-Hall, Englewood Cliffs, New Jersey

Bogdan R, Taylor S J 1975 Introduction to qualitative research methods: a phenomenological approach to the social sciences. Wiley, New York

Bottorff J L, Morse J M 1994 Identifying types of attending: patterns of nurses' work. Image: Journal of Nursing Scholarship 26(1): 53–60

Boud D 1987 A facilitator's view of adult learning. In: Boud D, Griffin V (eds) Appreciating adults learning: from the learners' perspective. Kogan Page, London, pp 222–239

Boud D, Keogh R, Walker D 1985 Reflection: turning experience into learning. Kogan Page, London

Boud D, Walker D 1990 Making the most of experience. Studies in Continuing Education 12(2): 61–80

Boydell T 1976 Experiential learning. Department of Adult and Higher Education, Manchester Monographs 5. University of Manchester, Manchester

Brookfield S D 1986 Understanding and facilitating adult learning. Open University Press, Milton Keynes

Brown J S, Tanner C A, Padrick K P 1984 Nursing's search for scientific knowledge. Nursing Research 33: 26–32

Brunner L S, Suddarth D S 1992 The textbook of adult nursing. Chapman Hall, London

Brykczynski K A 1989 An interpretative study describing the clinical judgment of nurse practitioners. Scholarly Inquiry for Nursing Practice: An International Journal 3(2): 75–104

Burgoyne J, Stuart R 1976 The nature, use and acquisition of managerial skills and other attributes. Personnel Review 5(4): 19–29

Burgoyne J G, Hodgson V E 1983 Natural learning and managerial action: a phenomenological study in the field setting. Journal of Management Studies 20(3): 387–399

Campbell M L 1984 Information systems and management in hospital nursing: a study in the social organization of knowledge. PhD thesis, Ontario Institute for Studies in Education, University of Toronto, Toronto

Campbell M L, Jackson N S 1992 Learning to nurse: plans, accounts and action. Qualitative Health Research 2(4): 475–496

Carper B A 1978 Fundamental patterns of knowing in nursing. Advances in Nursing Science 1(October): 13–23

Chené A 1985 Hermeneutics and the educational narrative. Proceedings of the Adult Education Research Conference, Tempe, Arizona. ERIC Microfiche

Chenitz W C, Swanson J M 1984 Surfacing nursing process: a method for generating nursing theory from practice. Journal of Advanced Nursing 9(7): 205–215

Chenitz W C, Swanson J M 1986 From practice to grounded theory: qualitative research in nursing. Addison-Wesley, Menlo Park

Chinn P L, Kramer M K 1995 Theory and nursing: a systematic approach, 4th edn. Mosby, Toronto

Choppin R G 1983 The role of the ward sister: a review of the British literature since 1967. King's Fund Project Paper 33. King Edward's Hospital Fund for London, London

Christman L 1985 Review of 'From novice to expert' by P Benner. Nursing Administration Quarterly 94: 87–89

Clandinin D J 1989 Developing rhythm in teaching: the narrative study of a beginning teacher's personal practical knowledge of classrooms. Curriculum Inquiry 19(2): 121–141

Clandinin D J, Connelly F M 1987 Teachers' personal knowledge: what counts as 'personal' in studies of the personal. Journal of Curriculum Studies 19(6): 487–500

Clark C L 1990 Theory and practice in social intervention: the case of voluntary action on unemployment. PhD thesis, University of Edinburgh, Edinburgh

Clark C L 1991 Theory and practice in voluntary social action. Avebury, Aldershot

Closs S J 1992 Patients' night-time pain, analgesic provision and sleep after surgery. International Journal of Nursing Studies 29(4): 381–392

Crabtree A, Jorgenson M 1986 Exploring the practical knowledge in expert critical care nursing practice. MScN thesis, University of Wisconsin — Madison

Darbyshire P 1994 Living with a sick child in hospital: the experiences of parents and nurses. Chapman & Hall, London

Davies J, Easterby-Smith M 1984 Learning and developing from managerial work experiences. Journal of Management Studies 21(2): 169–183

Denis M, Richter I 1987 Learning about intuitive learning: moose-hunting techniques. In: Boud D, Griffin V (eds) Appreciating adults learning: from the learners' perspective. Kogan Page, London, pp 25–36

Devine E C 1992 Effects of psycho-educational care for adult surgical patients: a meta-analysis of 191 studies. Patient Education and Counselling 19: 129–142

Dewey J 1925 Experience and nature. Open Court, Chicago

Dewey J 1938 Experience and education. Collier Books, New York

Dick J 1983 What makes an excellent practising nurse? Canadian Nurse 79(11): 44–47

Dickoff J, James P 1968 A theory of theories: a position paper. Nursing Research 17(3): 197–203

Dickoff J, James P 1975 Theory development in nursing. In: Verhonick P J (ed) Nursing research. Little, Brown & Company, Boston, pp 45–92

Diekelmann N 1989 The nursing curriculum: lived experiences of students. In: Curriculum revolution: reconceptualizing nursing education. National League for Nursing, New York, pp 25–41

Diekelmann N 1992 Learning-as-testing: a Heideggerian hermeneutical analysis of the lived experiences of students and teachers in nursing. Advances in Nursing Science 14(3): 72–83

Diekelmann N 1993 Behavioural pedagogy: a Heideggerian hermeneutical analysis of the lived experiences of students and teachers in baccalaureate nursing education. Journal of Nursing Education 32: 245–250

Diekelmann N, Allen D, Tanner C 1989 The NLN criteria for appraisal of baccalaureate programs: a critical hermeneutic analysis. National League for Nursing, New York

Dingwall R 1976 Accomplishing profession. In: Wadsworth

M, Robinson D (eds) Studies in everyday medical life. Martin Robertson, London, pp 91–107

Dreyfus H L 1980 Holism and hermeneutics. Review of Metaphysics 34(September): 3–23

Dreyfus H L 1983 Why current studies of human capacities can never be scientific. Berkeley Cognitive Science Report no 11. University of California at Berkeley

Dreyfus H 1987 Husserl, Heidegger and modern existentialism. In: Magee B (ed) The great philosophers. BBC Books, London, pp 252–277

Dreyfus H L 1991 Being-in-the-world: a commentary on Heidegger's 'Being and Time', Division 1. MIT Press, London

Dreyfus H L, Dreyfus S E 1986 Mind over machine: the power of human intuition and expertise in the era of the computer. The Free Press, New York

Dreyfus S E 1982 Formal models vs human situational understanding: inherent limitations on the modelling of business expertise. Office: Technology and People 1: 133–165

Duden B 1991 The woman beneath the skin: a doctor's patients in 18th-century Germany. Harvard University Press, Cambridge, Mass

Duffield C 1991 First-line nurse managers: issues in the literature. Journal of Advanced Nursing 16: 1247–1253

Dunn K, Schilder E 1993 Novice and expert head nurses: a comparative study of work activities and behaviours. Canadian Journal of Nursing Administration (March/April): 10–15

Elster S E 1987 An analysis of nurses who demonstrate clinical excellence in nursing. PhD dissertation, University of Utah

Emerson R M 1987 Four ways to improve the craft of fieldwork. Journal of Contemporary Ethnography 16(1): 69–89

Eraut M 1985 Knowledge creation and knowledge use in professional contexts. Studies in Higher Education 10(2): 117–133

Evers H 1982a Key issues in nursing practice: ward management — 1. Nursing Times Occasional Papers 78(6): 21–24

Evers H 1982b Key issues in nursing practice: ward management — 2. Nursing Times Occasional Papers 78(7): 25–26

Fagin C, Diers D 1984 Nursing as metaphor. International Nursing Review 31(1): 16–17

Fenton M V 1984 Identification of the skilled performance of master's prepared nurses as a method of curriculum planning and evaluation. In: Benner P From novice to expert: excellence and power in clinical nursing practice. Addison-Wesley, Menlo Park, California, pp 262–274

Fenton M V 1985 Identifying competencies of clinical nurse specialists. Journal of Nursing Administration 15(12): 31–37

Field P A 1980 An ethnography: four nurses' perspectives of nursing in a community setting. PhD thesis, University of Alberta

Field P A 1981 A phenomenological look at giving an injection. Journal of Advanced Nursing 6: 291–296

Field P A 1983 An ethnography: four public health nurses' perspectives of nursing. Journal of Advanced Nursing 8(1): 3–12

Fishbein E 1985 Intuition and intellectual education. The International Encyclopedia of Education, vol 5. Pergamon, London

Fitzpatrick J M, While A E, Roberts J 1992 The role of the nurse in high-quality patient care: a review of the literature. Journal of Advanced Nursing 17: 1210–1219

Flanagan J C 1954 The critical incident technique. Psychological Bulletin 51: 327–358

Ford J S 1989 Living with a history of a heart attack: a human science investigation. Journal of Advanced Nursing 14: 173–179

Fordham M 1988 Pain. In: Wilson-Barnett J, Batehup L (eds) Patient problems: a research base for nursing care. Scutari Press, London, pp 119–147

Forrest D 1989 The experience of caring. Journal of Advanced Nursing 14: 815–823

Freidson E 1986 Professional powers: a study of the institutionalization of formal knowledge. University of Chicago Press, Chicago

Freire P 1970 Pedagogy of the oppressed. Herder & Herder, New York

Fretwell J 1978 Socialisation of nurses: teaching and learning in hospital wards. PhD thesis, University of Warwick

Fretwell J 1982 Ward learning and teaching: sister and the learning environment. Royal College of Nursing, London

Gadamer H-G 1975 Truth and method. Sheed & Ward, London

Gadamer H-G 1979 The problem of historical consciousness. In: Rabinow P, Sullivan W M (eds) Interpretive social science, pp 103–160. University of California Press, Berkeley. (First published in Graduate Faculty Philosophy Journal 5(1), 1975)

Gadamer H-G 1981 Reason and the age of science. Translated by F G Lawrence. MIT Press, London

Garfinkel H 1967 Studies in ethnomethodology. Prentice-Hall, Englewood Cliffs, New Jersey

Geer B (ed) 1972 Learning to work. Sage, London

Giddens A 1976 New rules of sociological method. Hutchinson, London

Giddens A 1982 Profiles and critiques in social theory. Macmillan, London

Giorgi A 1975 An application of phenomenological method in psychology. In: Giorgi A, Fischer C, Murray C (eds) Duquesne studies in phenomenological psychology, vol 2. Duquesne University Press, Pittsburgh, pp 82–103

Giorgi A 1985 The phenomenological psychology of learning and the verbal learning tradition. In: Giorgi A (ed) Phenomenology and psychological research. Duquesne University Press, Pittsburgh, pp 23–85

Glaser B G 1978 Theoretical sensitivity. Scientific Press, Mill Valley, California

Glaser B G, Strauss A L 1967 The discovery of grounded theory: strategies for qualitative research. Aldine, New York

Glaser R 1987 Thoughts on expertise. In: Schooler C, Schaie K W (eds) Cognitive functioning and social structure over the life course. Ablex, Norwood, New Jersey, pp 81–94

Glass H 1983 Interventions in nursing: goal or task-oriented? International Nursing Review 30(2): 53–56

Goddard H A 1953 The work of nurses in hospital wards: report of a job-analysis. Nuffield Provincial Hospitals Trust, London

Gordon D R 1986 Models of clinical expertise in American nursing practice. Social Science and Medicine 22(9): 953–961

Gordon M 1985 Nursing diagnosis. In: Werley H H,

Fitzpatrick J J (eds) Annual review of nursing research. Springer, New York

Grant J, Marsden P 1988 Primary knowledge, medical education and consultant expertise. Medical Education 22: 173–179

Gray-Snelgrove R 1982 The experience of giving care to a parent dying of cancer: meanings identified through the process of shared reflection. PhD thesis, Ontario Institute for Studies in Education, University of Toronto

Griffin V R 1987 Naming the processes. In: Boud D, Griffin V (eds) Appreciating adults learning: from the learners' perspective. Kogan Page, London, pp 209–221

Griffin V R 1988 Learning to name our learning processes. Canadian Journal for the Study of Adult Education 2(2): 1–16

Gruber M, with Benner P 1989 A dialogue with excellence: the power of certainty. American Journal of Nursing (April): 502–503

Grypdonck M 1980 Theory and research in a practice discipline: the case of nursing. PhD thesis, University of Manchester

Grypdonck M 1987 The introduction of the nursing process in a home health agency. Paper presented at the International Nursing Research Congress, 29–30 July, Edinburgh

Guba E G, Lincoln Y S 1981 Effective evaluation. Jossey-Bass, San Francisco

Habermas J 1984 The theory of communicative action. Trans. T. McCarthy. Beacon Press, Boston

Hammer M, Champy J 1993 Re-engineering the corporation: a manifesto for business revolution. Harper Collins, New York

Hammersley M, Atkinson P 1983 Ethnography: principles in practice. Tavistock, London

Hasselkus B R, Ray R O 1988 Informal learning in family caregiving: a worm's eye view. Adult Education Quarterly 39(1): 31–40

Hayward J 1975 Information — a prescription against pain. Royal College of Nurses, London

Heidegger M 1962 Being and time. Translated by Macquarrie J, Robinson E. Basil Blackwood, Oxford

Henderson V 1966 The nature of nursing. Collier-Macmillan, London

Henderson V 1980 Preserving the essence of nursing in a technological age. Journal of Advanced Nursing 5: 245–260

Henry J 1989 Meaning and practice in experiential learning. In: Weil S, McGill I (eds) Making sense of experiential learning: diversity in theory and practice. Society for Research into Higher Education and Open University Press, Milton Keynes, pp 25–37

Hochschild A R 1983 The managed heart. University of California Press, Berkeley

Hodges L C, Knapp R, Cooper J 1987 Head nurses: their practice and education. Journal of Nursing Administration 17(12): 39–44

Holden G W, Klingner A M 1988 Learning from experience: differences in how novice vs. expert nurses diagnose why an infant is crying. Journal of Nursing Education 27(1): 23–29

Holm K, Cohen F, Dudas S et al 1989 Effects of personal pain experience on pain assessment. Image: Journal of Nursing Scholarship 21(2): 72–75

Honey M A 1987 The interview as text: hermeneutics considered as a model for analyzing the clinically informed research interview. Human Development 30(2): 69–82

Horvath K J, Secatore J A, Alpert H B, Costa M J, Powers E M, Stengrevics S S, Aroian J 1994 Uncovering the knowledge embedded in clinical nurse manager practice. Journal of Nursing Administration 7(8): 39–44

Hyslop A 1987 Clinical decision-making in nursing: can computers help? Paper presented at the Nursing Research Unit Seminar, Department of Nursing Studies, Edinburgh: University of Edinburgh

Inman U 1975 Towards a theory of nursing care. Royal College of Nursing and National Council of Nurses in the United Kingdom, London

Isenberg D J 1984 How senior managers think. Harvard Business Review (November-December): 81–90

Jacox A 1974 Theory construction in nursing: an overview. Nursing Research 23(1): 4–13

James C R, Clarke B A 1994 Reflective practice in nursing: issues and implications for nurse education. Nurse Education Today 14: 82–90

Jarvis P 1987a Adult learning in the social context. Croom Helm, London

Jarvis P 1987b Meaningful and meaningless experience: towards an analysis of learning from life. Adult Education Quarterly 37(3): 164–172

Jarvis P 1992 Paradoxes of learning: on becoming an individual in society. Jossey-Bass, San Francisco

Jenny J, Logan J 1992 Knowing the patient: one aspect of clinical knowledge. Image: Journal of Nursing Scholarship 24(4): 254–258

Johnson D E 1968 Theory in nursing: borrowed and unique. Nursing Research 17(3): 206–209

Johnson J E 1984 Coping with elective surgery. In: Werley H H, Fitzpatrick J J (eds) Annual review of nursing research, vol 2. Springer, New York, pp 107–132

Katz J 1988 Why doctors don't disclose uncertainty. In: Dowie J, Elstein A (eds) Professional judgment. Cambridge University Press, Cambridge, pp 544–565 (First published in Hastings Centre Report 14: 35–44, 1984)

Katzman E M, Roberts J I 1988 Nurse-physician conflicts as barriers to the enactment of nursing roles. Western Journal of Nursing Research 10(5): 576–590

Kennedy M 1983 Working knowledge. Knowledge: Creation, Diffusion, Utilization 5(2): 193–211

Kim M J 1989 Nursing diagnosis. In: Fitzpatrick J J, Taunton R L, Benoliel J Q (eds) Annual review of nursing research. Springer, New York, pp 117–142

Kitson A L 1986 Indicators of quality in nursing care — an alternative approach. Journal of Advanced Nursing 11: 133–144

Kitson A 1991 Therapeutic nursing and the hospitalised elderly. Scutari Press, London

Knafl K A, Webster D C 1988 Managing and analyzing qualitative data: a description of tasks, techniques, and materials. Western Journal of Nursing Research 10(2): 195–218

Knights S 1985 Reflection and learning: the importance of a listener. In: Boud D, Keogh R, Walker D (eds) Reflection: turning experience into learning. Kogan Page, London, pp 85–90

Kolb D 1984 Experiential learning: experience as the source of learning and development. Prentice-Hall, Englewood Cliffs, New Jersey

Kolb D A, Lewis L H 1986 Facilitating experiential learning: observations and reflections. In: Lewis L H (ed) Experiential and simulation techniques for teaching adults. New Directions for Continuing Education, no 30. Jossey-Bass, San Francisco

Kratz C R 1975 Participant observation in dyadic and triadic situations. International Journal of Nursing Studies 12: 169–174

Kuhn T S 1970 The structure of scientific revolutions, 2nd edn. University of Chicago Press, Chicago

Kuhn T S 1977 The essential tension. University of Chicago Press, Chicago

Larsson S 1986 Learning from experience: teachers' conceptions of changes in their professional practice. Journal of Curriculum Studies 19(1): 35–43

Lathlean J 1987 Job sharing a ward sister's post. A report of an evaluation commissioned by the Riverside Health Authority. Ashdale Press, Oxford

Lathlean J (ed) 1988 Research in action: developing the role of the ward sister. King's Fund Centre, London

Lathlean J, Farnish S 1984 The ward sister training project. Nursing Education Research Unit Report no 3. Department of Nursing Studies, Chelsea College, University of London, London

Lathlean J, Smith G, Bradley S 1986 Post-registration development schemes evaluation. Nursing Education Research Unit Report no. 4. Department of Nursing Studies, King's College, University of London, London

Le Breck D B 1989 Clinical judgment: a comparison of theoretical perspectives. In: Holzemer W L (ed) Review of research in nursing education. National League for Nursing, New York, pp 33–55

Lelean S R 1973 Ready for report nurse? A study of nursing communication in hospital wards. Royal College of Nursing, London

Lewin K 1952 Field theory in social science. Tavistock, London

Lewis T 1990 The hospital ward sister: professional gatekeeper. Journal of Advanced Nursing 15: 808–818

Llewelyn J 1985 Beyond metaphysics? The hermeneutic circle in contemporary Continental philosophy. Macmillan, London

Loomis M E 1985 Emerging content in nursing: an analysis of dissertation abstracts and titles: 1976–1982. Nursing Research 34(2): 113–118

McCall M W, Lombardo M M, Morrison A M 1988 The lessons of experience: how successful executives develop on the job. Lexington Books, Toronto

McFarlane J K 1970 The proper study of the nurse. Royal College of Nursing and National Council of Nurses of the United Kingdom, London

McFarlane J K 1976 A charter for caring. Journal of Advanced Nursing 1(3): 187–196

McFarlane J K 1977 Developing a theory of nursing: the relation of theory to practice, education and research. Journal of Advanced Nursing 2(3): 261–270

McFarlane of Llandaff Baroness J K 1989 Research, scholarship and practice. Paper presented at the Royal College of Nursing Research Society Conference, 14–16 April, Swansea, Wales

McFarlane of Llandaff Baroness J K, Castledine G 1982 A guide to the practice of nursing using the nursing process. C V Mosby, London

McGhee A 1961 The patient's attitude to nursing care. E & S Livingstone, Edinburgh

McGill I, Weil S 1990 Making sense of experiential learning.

Adults Learning 1(5): 136–139

McHugh N G, Christman N J, Johnson J E 1982 Preparatory information: what helps and why. American Journal of Nursing (May): 780–782

MacLeod M L P 1990 Experience in everyday nursing practice: a study of 'experienced' surgical ward sisters. PhD thesis, University of Edinburgh, Edinburgh

MacLeod M L P 1993 On knowing the patient: experiences of nurses undertaking care. In: Radley A (ed) Worlds of illness: biographical and cultural perspectives on health and disease. Routledge, London, pp 179–197

MacLeod M 1994 'It's the little things that count': the hidden complexity of everyday clinical nursing practice. Journal of Clinical Nursing 3(6): 361–368

MacLeod M L P 1995 What does it mean to be well taught? — A hermeneutic course evaluation. Journal of Nursing Education 34(5): 197–203

MacLeod M L P, Farrell P 1994 The need for significant reform: a practice-driven approach to curriculum. Journal of Nursing Education 33(5): 208–214

MacLeod Clark J 1982 Nurse-patient verbal interaction: an analysis of recorded conversations in selected surgical wards. PhD thesis, University of London

McWilliam C L, Wong C A 1994 Keeping it secret: the costs and benefits of nursing's hidden work in discharging patients. Journal of Advanced Nursing 19: 152–163

Magee B (ed) 1987 The great philosophers. BBC Books, London

Marsick V J, Watkins K E 1990 Informal and incidental learning in the workplace. Routledge, London

Marson S N 1981 Ward teaching skills — an investigation into the behavioural characteristics of effective ward teachers. MPhil thesis, Sheffield City Polytechnic

Marson S N 1982 Ward sister — teacher or facilitator? An investigation into the behavioural characteristics of effective ward sisters. Journal of Advanced Nursing 7: 347–357

Marton F, Hounsell D, Entwistle N 1984 The experience of learning. Scottish Academic Press, Edinburgh

May C 1990 Research on nurse-patient relationships: problems of theory, problems of practice. Journal of Advanced Nursing 15: 307–315

Mead G H 1934 Mind, self and society. University of Chicago Press, Chicago

Meleis A I 1987 Revisions in knowledge development: a passion for substance. Scholarly Inquiry for Nursing Practice: An International Journal 1(1): 5–19

Meleis A I 1991 Theoretical nursing: development and progress, 2nd edn. J B Lippincott, Philadelphia

Melia K M 1979 A sociological approach to the analysis of nursing work. Journal of Advanced Nursing 4: 57–67

Melia K M 1983 Doing nursing and being professional. Nursing Times (June 1): 28–30

Melia K M 1987 Learning and working: the occupational socialization of nurses. Tavistock, London

Merleau-Ponty M 1962 The phenomenology of perception. Translated by Smith C. Routledge & Kegan Paul, London

Merriam S B 1987 Adult learning and theory building: a review. Adult Education Quarterly 37(4): 187–198

Mezirow J 1981 A critical theory of adult learning and education. Adult Education 32(1): 3–24

Mezirow J 1990 Fostering critical reflection in adulthood. Jossey-Bass, San Francisco

Mezirow J 1994 Understanding transformation theory. Adult Education Quarterly 44(4): 222–232

Moore D T 1986 Learning at work: case studies in non-school education. Anthropology and Education Quarterly 17: 166–184

Moores Y 1989 Some issues for nursing practice in the 1990s. Paper presented at New Directions for Clinical Nursing, the RCN Hartlepool Branch/Nursing Standard eighth national conference, Hartlepool, England

Moult A P, Melia K M, Hockey L 1978 Patterns of ward organization. Report for the Leverhulme Trust. Nursing Research Unit, University of Edinburgh, Edinburgh

Mueller-Vollmer K (ed) 1985 The hermeneutics reader: texts of the German tradition from the Enlightenment to the present. Basil Blackwell, Oxford

Munhall P L, Oiler Boyd C J 1993 Nursing research: a qualitative perspective, 2nd edn. National League for Nursing, New York

National Board for Scotland 1989 Preparation for practice: nursing and midwifery education — papers for comment (1992 programmes). National Board for Nursing, Midwifery and Health Visiting for Scotland, Edinburgh

Nisbett R E, Wilson D W 1977 Telling more than we can know: verbal reports on mental processes. Psychological Review 84(3): 231–259

Norman I J, Redfern S J, Tomalin D A, Oliver S 1994 Kitson's Therapeutic Nursing Function Indicator as a predictor of the quality of nursing care in hospital wards. International Journal of Nursing Studies 31(2): 109–118

O'Brien B, Pearson A 1993 Unwritten knowledge in nursing: consider the spoken as well as the written word. Scholarly Inquiry for Nursing Practice: An International Journal 7(2): 111–124

Ogier M E 1982 An ideal sister? A study of the leadership style and verbal interactions of ward sisters with nurse learners in general hospitals. Royal College of Nursing, London

Ogier M 1986 An 'ideal' sister — seven years on. Nursing Times Occasional Paper 82(2): 54–57

Oiler C 1982 The phenomenological approach in nursing research. Nursing Research 31(3): 178–181

Olsen S 1985 Exploring the clinical practice of expert oncology nurses. MScN thesis, University of Wisconsin — Madison

Omery A 1983 Phenomenology: a method for nursing research. Advances in Nursing Science (January): 49–63

Orton H 1979 Ward learning climate and student nurse response. MPhil thesis, Sheffield City Polytechnic

Orton H 1981 Ward learning climate: a study of the role of the ward sister in relation to student learning on the ward. Royal College of Nursing, London

Packer M J 1985 Hermeneutic inquiry in the study of human conduct. American Psychologist 40(10): 1081–1093

Palmer R E 1969 Hermeneutics. Northwestern University Press, Evanston

Parker J, Gardner G, Wiltshire J 1992 Handover: the collective narrative of nursing practice. Australian Journal of Advanced Nursing 9(3): 31–37

Pembrey S 1980 The ward sister — key to nursing. Royal College of Nursing, London

Pembrey S 1989 The development of nursing practice: a new contribution. Senior Nurse 9(8): 3–8

Pirsig R M 1974 Zen and the art of motorcycle maintenance. Bantam Books, New York

Polanyi M [1958]1962 Personal knowledge. Routledge & Kegan Paul, London

Polanyi M 1966 The tacit dimension. Routledge & Kegan Paul, London

Polkinghorne D 1988 Narrative knowing and the human sciences. State University of New York Press, Albany

Prescott P A, Dennis K E, Jacox A K 1987 Clinical decision making of staff nurses. Image: Journal of Nursing Scholarship 19(2): 56–62

Pyles S H, Stern P N 1983 Discovery of nursing gestalt in critical care nursing: the importance of the Gray Gorilla Syndrome. Image: The Journal of Nursing Scholarship 15(2): 51–57

Rabinow P, Sullivan W M 1979 Interpretative social science. University of California Press, Berkeley

Rather M 1992 Nursing as a way of thinking — A Heideggerian hermeneutical analysis of the lived experience of the returning Registered Nurse. Research in Nursing and Health 15: 47–55

Redfern S 1981 Hospital sisters: their job attitudes and occupational stability. Royal College of Nursing, London

Revans R W 1964 Standards for morale: cause and effect in hospitals. Oxford University Press for the Nuffield Provincial Hospitals Trust, London

Revans R W 1980 Action learning. Blond & Briggs, London

Rew L 1986 Intuition: concept analysis of a group phenomenon. Advances in Nursing Science 8(2): 21–28

Ricoeur P 1978 The task of hermeneutics. In: Murray M (ed) *Heidegger and modern philosophy*. Yale University Press, New Haven, pp 141–160 (First published in Philosophy Today 17(Summer), 1973)

Ricoeur P 1979 The model of the text: meaningful action considered as text. In: Rabinow P, Sullivan W M (eds) Interpretative social science. University of California Press, Berkeley, pp 73–101 (First published in Social Research 38(3), 1971)

Rittman M, Northsea C, Hausauer N, Green C, Swanson L 1993 Living with renal failure. ANNA Journal 20(3): 327–332

Roach Sr S M 1987 The human act of caring. The Canadian Hospital Association, Ottawa

Robinson C A, Thorne S E 1988 Dilemmas of ethics and validity in qualitative nursing research. Canadian Journal of Nursing Research 20(1): 65–76

Robinson J, Elkan R 1989. Research for policy and policy for research: A review of selected DHSS commissioned nurse education research 1975–1986. Nursing Policy Studies Centre, University of Warwick, Coventry

Rogers J, Powell D 1983 The career patterns of nurses who have completed a Joint Board of Clinical Nursing Studies certificate. Report of the follow-up study, vol. 1. Department of Health and Social Services, Joint Board of Clinical Nursing Studies, London

Rogers M E 1970 An introduction to the theoretical basis of nursing. Davis, Philadelphia

Rossing B 1991 Patterns of informal incidental learning: insights from community action. International Journal of Lifelong Education 10(1): 45–60

Rossing B, Russell R 1987 Informal adult experiential learning: reality in search of a theory and a practice. In: Rivera W M, Walker S M (eds) Lifelong learning research conference proceedings, College Park, Maryland, pp 158–162

Royal College of Nursing 1980 Standards of nursing care: a discussion document. Royal College of Nursing, London

Royal College of Nursing 1981 Towards standards: a discussion document. Royal College of Nursing, London

Runciman P J 1983 Ward sister at work. Churchill Livingstone, Edinburgh

Ryle G 1949 The concept of mind. Hutchinson's University Library, London

Sacks O 1985 The man who mistook his wife for a hat. Duckworth, London

Sanday P R 1979 The ethnographic paradigm(s). Administrative Science Quarterly 24(4): 527–538

Schilder E 1986 The use of physical restraints on an acute care medical ward. DNSc dissertation, University of California, San Francisco

Schilder E 1989 Bodily perceptions and their influence on health. Nursing Standard 4(13/14): 30–32

Schön D A 1983 The reflective practitioner: how professionals think in action. Basic Books, New York

Schön D A 1987 Educating the reflective practitioner. Jossey-Bass, San Francisco

Schutz A, Luckmann T 1974 Structures of the life-world. Heinemann, London

Scribner S 1986 Thinking in action: some characteristics of practical thought. In: Sternberg R J, Wagner R K (eds) Practical intelligence. Cambridge University Press, Cambridge, pp 13–30

Seers C J 1987 Pain, anxiety and recovery in patients undergoing surgery. PhD thesis, King's College, University of London

Selman M 1988 Learning and philosophy of mind. Canadian Journal for the Study of Adult Education 2(2): 28–42

Senge P M 1990 The fifth discipline: the art and practice of the learning organization. Doubleday, New York

Silverman D 1989 Telling convincing stories: a plea for cautious positivism in case studies. In: Glassner B, Moreno J D (eds) The qualitative-quantitative distinction in the social sciences. Kluwer Academic, Dordrecht, pp 57–77

Smith P A 1988 Quality of nursing and the ward as a learning environment for student nurses: a multi-method approach. PhD thesis, University of London

Smith P 1992 The emotional labour of nursing — how nurses care. Macmillan, London

Spiegelberg H 1982 The phenomenological movement: a historical introduction, 3rd edn. Martinus Nijhoff, The Hague

Stainton M C 1992 Mismatched caring in high-risk perinatal situations. Clinical Nursing Research 1(1): 35–49

Steele S, Fenton M V 1988 Expert practice of clinical nurse specialists. Clinical Nurse Specialist 2(1): 45–52

Strauss A, Fagerhaugh S, Suczek B, Wiener C 1985 Social organization of medical work. University of Chicago Press, Chicago

Street A F 1992 Inside nursing: a critical ethnography of clinical nursing practice. State University of New York Press, Albany

Strong P M 1979 The ceremonial order of the clinic. Routledge & Kegan Paul, London

Tanner C A 1983 Research on clinical judgment. In: Holzemer W L (ed) Review of research in nursing education. Slack, New Jersey, pp 2–32

Tanner C A 1987 Teaching clinical judgment. In: Fitzpatrick J J, Taunton R L (eds) Annual review of nursing research. Springer, New York, pp 153–173

Tanner C A 1989 Use of research in clinical judgment. In: Tanner C A, Lindeman C A (eds) Using nursing research. National League for Nursing, New York, pp 19–34

Tanner C A, Benner P, Chesla C, Gordon D R 1993 The phenomenology of knowing the patient. Image: Journal of Nursing Scholarship 25(4): 273–280

Taylor B 1994 Being human: ordinariness in nursing. Churchill Livingstone, Melbourne

Taylor C 1971 Interpretation and the sciences of man. Review of Metaphysics 25(1): 1–51 (Also in Taylor C 1985 Philosophy and the human sciences. Philosophical papers 2. Cambridge University Press, Cambridge)

Taylor C 1985 Theories of meaning. In: Human agency and language. Philosophical papers 1. Cambridge University Press, Cambridge

Taylor M 1986 Learning for self-direction in the classroom: the pattern of a transitional process. Studies in Higher Education 11(1): 55–72

Taylor M 1987 Self-directed learning: more than meets the observer's eye. In: Boud D, Griffin V (eds) Appreciating adults learning: from the learners' perspective. Kogan Page, London, pp 179–196

Thomas A M 1986 Review of adult learning: research and practice, by H E Long. Learning (Canadian Association for Adult Education) 4(3): 21–22

Thorne S E, Robinson C A 1988 Reciprocal trust in health care relationships. Journal of Advanced Nursing 13: 782–789

Tilley S 1995 Negotiating realities: making sense of interaction between patients diagnosed as neurotic and nurses. Avebury, Aldershot

Tough A 1979 The adult's learning projects, 2nd edn. Ontario Institute for Studies in Education, Toronto

Tough A 1982 Intentional changes: a fresh approach to helping people change. Follett, Chicago

United Kingdom Central Council 1986 Project 2000: a new preparation for practice. United Kingdom Central Council for Nursing, Midwifery and Health Visiting, London

United Kingdom Central Council 1990 Discussion paper on post-registration education and practice. Post-registration Education and Practice Project (PREPP). United Kingdom Central Council for Nursing, Midwifery and Health Visiting, London

United Kingdom Department of Health and Social Services 1986 Report of the Nursing Process Evaluation Working Group to the DHSS Nursing Research Liaison Group. [Chairman, Dame P Friend] Nursing Education Research Unit Report no 5. Department of Nursing Studies, King's College, University of London, London

United Kingdom Ministry of Health, Department of Health for Scotland and Ministry of Labour and National Service 1947. Report of the Working Party on the Recruitment and Training of Nurses. [Chairman, R S Wood] HMSO, London

United Kingdom Ministry of Health and Scottish Home and Health Department 1966 Report of the Committee on Senior Nursing Staff Structure. [Chairman, Sir B Salmon] HMSO, London

United Kingdom Parliament 1972 Report of the Committee on Nursing. [Chairman, Professor A Briggs] Cmnd 5115. HMSO, London

United Kingdom Parliament 1979 Report of the Royal Commission on the National Health Service. [Chairman, Sir A Merrison] Cmnd 7615. HMSO, London

Usher R 1992 Experience in adult education: a post-modern critique. Journal of Philosophy of Education 26(2): 201–214

Van Kaam A L 1959 Phenomenal analysis: exemplified by a

study of the experience of 'really feeling understood'. Journal of Individual Psychology 15: 66–72

Van Manen M 1984 Practising phenomenological writing. Phenomenology + Pedagogy 2(1): 36–69

Van Manen M 1989 By the light of anecdote. Phenomenology + Pedagogy 7: 232–253

Van Velsor E, Hughes M 1990. Gender differences in the development of managers: how women managers learn from experience. Technical report number 145, Center for Creative Leadership, Greensboro, North Carolina

Visintainer M A 1986 The nature of knowledge and theory in nursing. Image: Journal of Nursing Scholarship 182(Summer): 32–38

Watkins K E, Marsick V J 1992 Towards a theory of informal and incidental learning in organizations. International Journal of Lifelong Education 11(4): 287–300

Watkins K E, Marsick V J 1993 Sculpting the learning organization. Jossey-Bass, San Francisco

Webb C 1984 A nursing study of recovery from hysterectomy. PhD thesis, University of London

Webb C 1986 Professional and lay support for hysterectomy patients. Journal of Advanced Nursing 11: 167–177

Weber S J 1986 The nature of interviewing. Phenomenology

& Pedagogy 4(2): 65–72

Wilkinson C, Peters L, Mitchell K, Irwin T, McCorrie K, MacLeod M 1995 'Being there': an active approach to learning. Manuscript submitted for publication

Williams D 1969 The administrative contribution of the nursing sister. Public Administration 47: 307–328

Williams S 1989 The Radcliffe revolution. Nursing Times 85(18): 51–53

Wilson-Barnett J 1988 Nursing values: exploring the clichés. Journal of Advanced Nursing 13: 790–796

Wilson-Barnett J, Batehup L 1988 Patient problems: a research base for nursing care. Scutari Press, London

Wilson-Barnett J, Fordham M 1982 Recovery from illness. John Wiley & Sons, Chichester

Working Party on Continuing Education 1981 Continuing education for the nursing profession in Scotland. [Chairman: M Auld] Edinburgh

Wros P L 1993 Behind the curtain: nursing care of dying patients in critical care. Unpublished PhD dissertation. Oregon Health Science University, Oregon

Wros P L 1994 The ethical context of nursing care of dying patients in critical care. In: Benner P (ed) Interpretative phenomenology: embodiment, caring, and ethics in health and illness. Sage, London

Index